The Womanly Art
of
Breastfeeding

La Leche League
Louise Arsenault 774-3722
Box 561
WINCHESTER, Ontario   K0C 2K0

$3.50 Softcover

$5.00 Hardcover

The Womanly Art
of
Breastfeeding

Foreword by
Herbert Ratner, M.D.

Drawings by
Joy Sidor

LA LECHE LEAGUE INTERNATIONAL
FRANKLIN PARK, ILLINOIS

First edition, September, 1958
17,000 copies
Second edition (revised and enlarged), May, 1963
PRINTINGS
First, 10,000, May, 1963
Second, 10,000, October, 1963
Third, 10,000, March, 1964
Fourth, 10,000, September, 1964
Fifth, 10,000, April, 1965
Sixth, 10,000, December, 1965
Seventh, 15,700, July, 1966
Eighth, 25,000, January, 1967
Ninth, 25,000, February, 1968
Tenth, 35,000, November, 1968
Eleventh, 40,000, October, 1969
Twelfth, 40,000, May, 1970
Thirteenth, 50,000, April, 1971
Fourteenth, 50,000, April, 1972
Fifteenth, 50,000, December, 1972
Sixteenth, 50,000, July, 1973
Seventeenth, 55,000, April, 1974
Eighteenth, 52,500, December, 1974
Nineteenth, 53,000, July, 1975
Twentieth, 53,000, January, 1976
Twenty-First, 50,000, June, 1976
Twenty-Second, 54,000, October, 1976
Twenty-Third, 54,000, July, 1977
Copyright 1958 and 1963 by La Leche League International
Hardcover   ISBN 0-912500-00-X
Softcover   ISBN 0-912500-01-8
Library of Congress Card Number:
63-14460
Printed in the U.S.A.
by Interstate Printers and Publishers, Inc.

Foreword

It was the famous Dr. Oliver Wendell Holmes who, in an address before the Massachusetts Medical Society in 1860, first pointed out for our times the unsuspectedly close "relation between the medical sciences and the conditions of society and the general thought of the time." He knew that "theoretically medicine ought to go on its own straightforward inductive path without regard . . . . to fluctuations of public opinion," but he was candid enough to recognize the great sensitivity "of medicine, professedly founded on observation, to outside influences."

Nowhere has the effect of outside influences been more obvious than in the steady decline of breastfeeding in the United States. Physicians know that breastfeeding is best. Oliver Wendell Holmes himself made this unequivocally clear when he stated as an eternal truth, with all of the backing of nature's long history and wisdom, that "a pair of substantial mammary glands has the advantage over the two hemispheres of the most learned professor's brain, in the art of compounding a nutritious fluid for infants." Yet, despite what the experience, art and science of medicine teaches them in no uncertain terms, most physicians have stood by —more or less as innocent bystanders—while the vagaries of women, the styles of the time, and cultural pressures have converted the preferred and the customary into the exceptional, with much disservice to mother and baby alike.

This insidious progression is understandable. Physicians are human beings and patients their partners in the therapeutic decision. Physicians cannot be expected to stand up, day after day, to the pressures of women who, uncertain and misinformed about breastfeeding themselves, are confused by conflicting voices as to what they should do. These include the voices of cousins and aunts, mothers and in-laws, girl friends, nurses, and others. Society and the women in their lives (and the men) are not impressing upon them the positive values of breastfeeding nor the opportunity they have for fulfilling themselves as women through nursing. Rather they keep suggesting the illusive simplicity of technologically proven, withal impersonalized, bottle feeding for nursing. Meanwhile, all are barraged by seductive advertisements from formula manufacturers lauding the new imitations. None speak up for Nature, Inc., which offers the original— the only natural food uniquely designed for human infants— with its backing of thousands of centuries of evolutionary perfection and truly long-term clinical success.

It is clear that physicians cannot fight this battle alone. That is why physicians are most grateful to La Leche League, which has dedicated itself to the recovery of Nature's womanly art of breastfeeding. It carries with it the hope of rescuing us from a sick technological age by the restoration of certain basic human relations leading to a more wholesome culture.

Several things should be known about La Leche League.

1. They have placed themselves from the beginning under the continuing supervision of physicians.

2. They see themselves as assistant to the medical profession in the goal of achieving the optimum nurturing of newborns by helping mothers rediscover motherhood in its fullness.

3. Recognizing the dangers of proselytizing and that example is the best educator and that success and its rewards are contagious, they have restricted their activity to women who have expressed a desire to nurse their babies.

4. They have not confused or prostituted their goal as a voluntary lay health organization by seeking financial support from the public.

5. More significant than all for society, they are seeking —by supporting mothers in this important early decision of motherhood—to help women to know themselves, to know the nature of womanly work, to know the critical contribution of woman to stable family life, and to help women become exemplars of dedication to duty with joy as a reward.

6. Finally, they recognize with Gilbert K. Chesterton, as expressed in his famous passage from *What's Wrong with the World*, that the career of a mother within the home is vaster than the career seeking of a woman away from the home.

> To be Queen Elizabeth within a definite area, deciding sales, banquets, labors, and holidays; to be Whiteley within a certain area, providing toys, boots, sheets, cakes and books; to be Aristotle within a certain area, teaching morals, manners, theology and hygiene: I can understand how this might exhaust the mind, but I cannot imagine how it could narrow it. How can it be a large career to tell other people's children about the Rule of Three and a small career to tell one's own children about the universe? How can it be broad to be the same thing to everyone, and narrow to be everything to someone? No; a woman's function is laborious but because it is gigantic, not because it is minute.

Lastly, as a physician who specializes in community health, I believe the following can be said. In an age when the indices to a sick society are high—mental illness, psychosomatic disease, suicide, delinquency, alcoholism, drug addiction, illegitimacy, divorce, etc.—we can only give support to an organization which strives, by prescribing the script prepared for mothers by Nature, to return them to their fundamental role of preserving the total health of the healthy newborn. When breasts lose their prime function, we have a distortion in society. Furthermore, since postpartum functioning breasts have an homeostatic and reciprocal relation to the infant, it should not be too much of a strain on our biological backgrounds to recognize that nonfunctioning breasts may lead in subtle ways to poorly functioning infants.

As confirmatory of the good work of La Leche League, I am also happy to report that many family physicians, pediatricians, and obstetricians have found their written materials, their classes, and their personal follow-up in support of individual nursing mothers of great value in their practice.

HERBERT RATNER, M.D.

Director
Oak Park Department of Public Health
Oak Park, Illinois

This is a simple story about a simple, normal function. Mothers have happily nursed their babies since the time of Eve. Breastfeeding is a natural and unique system of supply and demand which best serves mother and baby. Breastfeeding has not become complicated; only our attitudes toward it have created problems. It was to help solve these problems that *The Womanly Art of Breastfeeding* was written.

Contents

CHAPTER

Chapter 1

Best for Baby—Best for You

You are a woman who seeks to learn the ways of mothering through breastfeeding. You have never been more aware of your womanliness. You're going to have a baby, and you find it at once unbelievable and the focus of all your thoughts. Your body quietly holds the new life, faithfully serves it. Alternately your mind struggles between reverential awe and half-admitted reluctance. It is still so indistinct, so much only "it," but created in love and for eternity, a part of you. Fit him into your heart, you decide, and he will fit into your life.

You go to your doctor, and he makes his confirmation, "Healthy, happy, and pregnant." Hopefully, intently, you wait. Then you feel the flutter, the unmistakable stirring deep in your body. Life! Exciting, joyful, this revelation of the soul of your child.

Days follow each other, adding strength to the child and bringing increased changes in your body. More and more you're aware of the expanding cradle of your body, the swelling readiness of your breasts. You tire more easily, but carry yourself tall and proud, as on the day you were a bride. Beautiful and cherished as the tree heavy with fruit, you accept the waiting.

Six, seven, eight months. Patient months. A time of watchfulness and extra care. And a time to learn, to prepare yourself for your part in the coming birth. Your own special de-

1

light is gathering baby clothes, fixing a bassinet, musing on a name. Will it be a boy or girl?

Then when you least expect it, after such a long time of "expecting," you feel the twinge. And another. The time is here. Mingled relief and anticipation work a catch in your throat and you're thankful for the last-minute preparations. You wonder at your own emotions, at the shadow of fearfulness in your heart. Nature allows no turning back, and what woman, so blessed, would want to? Today your baby will be born!

Now you're impatient of the preliminary routine, anxious to settle down to the work of giving birth. And you're very grateful for the pressure of your husband's strong hand in yours. A wonderful father, you think, and then your consciousness centers on the process working within you. Rhythmically the birth force rises, swells as a great sea wave, peaks and recedes. Inexorably your body takes command. You will your muscles to cooperate, and in the calm interims, you rest satisfied.

The tempo quickens. This life will be, will be. The contractions break, crash hard, leave you tired, discouraged. From beyond the lights you hear the steady voice of your doctor. "Soon you will have a baby. You're doing a fine job." Reassured, strengthened, you breathe deeply and with control. And you work! Labor is a fitting term. The next moment is the bursting forth of blessed birth! You gasp for air and hear his cry. Was a sound ever before so priceless? Your heart pounds a prayer and your whole being reaches out to him. He was so long a part of you, he belongs close still. How vulnerable he looks, how indignant, how wonderful!

At last, quivering, he is placed in your arms. You hold him gloriously close, kiss his cheek, stroke his damp hair. Possessive love trembles through you. Again your body cradles him. You offer the full roundness of your breast. He sleeps! No matter. This has been a busy day. And there is time. Time to grow and to learn together. You'll begin again the patient months. You wonder that so great a part of the world is in such a rush. In a rush to send each of you on your separate ways, and in a rush to rationalize your loss. You wonder that mankind, preoccupied as it is with adjustment-making, can so regularly ignore the first to be faced. Only minutes before the umbilical cord was cut. Who is to snatch up your newborn, bridge the change of worlds, soothe and secure? Strangers?

He stirs, whimpers, declaring the import of the moment. Gently you stroke his cheek. He turns and nuzzles your

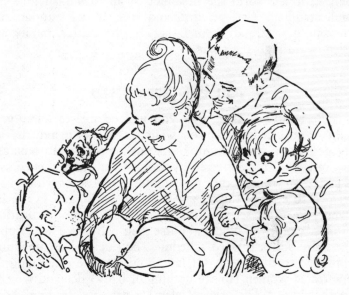

Of course you can nurse your baby

breast. Quickly you form the nipple with your fingers, a small help for one so little. His tiny mouth grasps and he sucks. Together you relax. What a kind, knowing Nature to demand so little now. Your tired body is not taxed. After the supreme effort of giving birth, this is sweet reward. And in good time, you know, with no thought on your part, the milk will come.

You look beyond to the steady repetition of days at the breast. The security of your arms, the soft warmth of your breast, the ready comfort of your milk, the quieting pulse of your body—all precious food to fill out his body, quicken his soul. You are so at peace. Is not this the ageless beauty of Madonna and Child, a time full of grace?

You hug him to you, fiercely aware of his dependence on you. Of course he will grow, will reach out, leave you. But not today. Give us time, you plead, let there be no regrets. Let us secure a new cord, one plaited simply and naturally of our constant closeness and many unhurried days. Not to be cut, it will form the first link of all to human love and understanding. And set firm and true, it will support and entwine new strands from father, brother, sister, family and friends, through the years.

YOU CAN BREASTFEED

Be reassured, then, that you will be able to nurse your baby. You can because you want to. But—is merely having the desire to nurse enough? Breastfeeding is basically a natural art, or should be, possessed by woman and strengthened as it is passed on from mother to daughter. Time and customs have seemed to change this in our modern world, and in the last twenty years we seem to have ignored the natural inclinations of most women to hold and nurse their baby. We have tipped the baby scales toward schedules, bottles, and an unnatural approach to the infant. Of late, however, the grumblings of unsatisfied women (to say nothing of baby) demand we take another look. "The original plan for care and feeding" bears re-examination. Many forward-looking doctors are taking a backward glance and realizing the unique good of breast-feeding and recommending it.

This is where we come in. We are friends who believe we can help you because we have all successfully nursed our babies and have helped others. It hasn't always been clear sailing, though. We can understand the worries and doubts of the inexperienced mother, since not all of us achieved complete success the first time. We are eager to share our experiences with you. As a beginning, here is this book. Maybe it will be all you need, especially if you are lucky enough to have the admiration and encouragement of someone near to you. If you have to go it alone for the time being, look us up in the section in the back of the book, "About La Leche League," and know that we are always ready to personally give you whatever help you need.

Let's stop a minute here, to see why things get so "out of hand." Why was this wonderful, womanly art so nearly lost? What caused the switch-over to bottles and formula when Nature's way had survived and thrived for centuries? How did Eve manage? Certainly she didn't join a league. Eve had it easy. Her baby came; the milk came; she nursed her baby. No well-meaning but not too well-informed friends questioned her ability to do this; it was simply taken for granted, like her ability to walk.

Also, Eve had no choice to confuse her. There just weren't any bottles and formulas. Now the bottles and formulas we have today are a good substitute, no doubt about it. The medical profession, in its role of assisting or substituting for Nature, tackled the problem of finding an acceptable milk for the occasional baby who could not get breast milk. With the help of refrigeration, sterilization, and the rubber company, the modern formula was delivered. It worked, and though still only a substitute, like crutches, it was better than nothing in the exceptional case.

Then, somehow, the exception became the rule. It was as though crutches became so fashionable that a pair was routinely issued to each and every person, without bothering to inquire whether or not they were needed. But, you may ask, why on earth did the medical profession begin prescribing these formulas right and left when they knew that, unlike the crutches, the formulas were seldom really needed? It wasn't as simple as that, of course; these things really did become needed, more and more, because a kind of vicious circle was set up.

You see, bottle feeding led gradually to a whole new way of bringing up babies. So many new decisions had to be made; which formula to use, how to prepare it, how much, whether you should hold the baby or not, and if so, how long—a mother could easily begin to regard her baby as a most complex digestive system instead of a dependent person with feelings of his own. Bogged down in scales and charts and schedules, mothers began to lose confidence in their own abilities, and often missed the easy, natural enjoyment of a

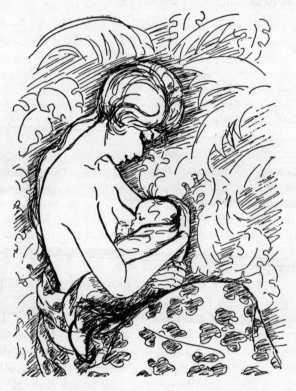

Eve just did what came naturally

new baby. Imagine, too, their loss of confidence, perplexity, and perhaps complete failure of breastfeeding if it were constantly being questioned and criticized. The physical reasons why a mother would be unable to nurse her baby are rare. (We mention them briefly on page 52).

Knowing these things, then, and knowing that you can get the help and encouragement you need, you will be able to say, "Yes, I can breastfeed my baby."

WHY YOU SHOULD BREASTFEED

BEST FOR BABY

Breast Milk Is Superior Infant Food

No one has ever proved otherwise, and we are confident no one ever will. The highest praise a formula manufacturer can give his product is that it is "most like mother's milk" or "nearer to mother's milk." Note that he cannot claim that it is better than, or even just as good as, mother's milk. The best he can claim is that it is "most like" or "nearer to" the product he considers the best, to which there is nothing superior.

Human milk, being form fitted to the human baby's digestive system, is more readily assimilated than cow's milk (which explains, incidentally, why most breastfed babies are fed more often than formula-fed babies). Because it is easier to digest, the baby's energy is conserved for better growth of his brain and body—an important consideration during the early months, when the rate of growth is far greater than at any other period of his life.

Mother's milk cannot be duplicated because we still do not know all the components of breast milk. Some years ago a well-known and widely-used infant formula was causing convulsions in a certain number of babies. The reason for this was found to be the lack of Vitamin B-6 in the formula. No one had known previously that this vitamin was needed by infants. Periodically the formula manufacturers find additional elements to be added. So any substitute, even though composed of all the things now known to be needed, may well be lacking in some essential factor not yet discovered in human milk.

Another consideration of some importance in this atomic age is the presence in milk of such products of radioactive fallout as strontium-90. The harmful effects of ionizing radiation are said to be greater, the younger the child. The consensus of scientific thought is that the amount of such radiation-emitting bodies present in breast milk is significantly smaller than that found in formula milk. Since milk makes up the greatest part of the infant's diet for some months, this may be a critical factor in modern times.

It should also be mentioned that in case of any major disaster which disrupts the supply services (water, milk, electricity, and so on) and perhaps contaminates food supplies on hand, a baby's survival may well depend on whether or not he is breastfed.

Allergies

Authorities state that mother's milk itself never causes allergic reactions, such as eczema, in a baby. Such allergies do occur with breast-milk substitutes with relatively high frequency. Many difficulties, some severe, extend beyond infancy. How often have you heard a mother remark, sometimes rather proudly, "Such-and-such didn't agree with Johnny; the doctor had to prescribe *three* (or maybe *four*, or even *five*) different formulas before he found one that agreed with him." Meanwhile, poor Johnny!

Allergic reactions to artificial food can be so severe that they actually threaten the life of a baby. When this happens, sometimes the only way the doctors can save the baby's life is by giving him breast milk from other mothers.

Breastfed Babies Are Healthier

We who nurse our babies have often been agreeably surprised to note that when the rest of the family comes down with a cold or flu, the baby remains free of it, or has only a mild case. Studies have shown that breastfeeding definitely prolongs the period of natural immunity to virus diseases. These include mumps, measles, polio, some kinds of pneumonia and other respiratory infections, and some diarrhea. In a study once made of twenty thousand babies under one year, it was found that there were twice as many infections in the bottle-fed infants as in the breastfed; ten times as many died from infections. This study was made before the days of antibiotics, so perhaps the percentages would be different now. But prevention is still safer and better than cure, and it should be noted that the antibiotics are of no use in combatting most virus diseases, that harmful side-effects do sometimes occur, and that some kinds of germs which once succumbed quickly are now becoming increasingly resistant to most antibiotics.

In the special case of the premature infant, doctors have pointed out the great importance of breast milk, and have especially stressed the value of colostrum, the fluid which is secreted before the true milk comes in. Colostrum contains five or six times as much protein as the later milk and only half as much fat and carbohydrates, which are not as easily digested by the newborn, premature baby, and undoubtedly other unknown properties.

In short, no formulas will ever be *better* than breast milk. And no matter how nearly science is able to approximate breast milk, the importance of breastfeeding in the mother-child relationship remains.

BEST FOR MOTHER
Gets You Back into Shape

Putting the newborn baby to the breast as soon as possible after birth helps to control blood loss. The baby's sucking causes the uterus to contract, which helps prevent hemorrhage after delivery. Also, continued nursing will help you to get back into shape again internally.

Breast Cancer

Many studies indicate that nursing your baby will improve your chances of avoiding breast cancer. Other studies conclude that it makes no difference; but in these the duration and type of breastfeeding apparently were not taken into account. Cancer of the breast is rare in areas of the world where prolonged breastfeeding is practiced, and this fact supports the studies indicating that women who nurse their babies as Nature intended are less likely to develop breast cancer.

Natural Spacing

Studies have shown that complete breastfeeding (no solids or supplements) for the first four to six months also has a definite effect on the natural spacing of children, since it usually tends to postpone the resumption of ovulation and the menstrual cycle for seven to fifteen months. The babies are then usually born about two years apart. It is *not* true that you cannot become pregnant as long as you are nursing, but pregnancy is extremely unusual before the first menstrual period, if you are *completely* nursing your baby. This means extra time in which to enjoy and pay special attention to your baby before the next comes along—and extra time for the baby to develop the security that comes from undivided maternal attention.

Gift of Time and Money

An intangible, but very real, bonus to the nursing mothers is the gift of time. This includes hours *not* spent in preparing, sterilizing, warming, cooling, and cleaning up after formula (these seem like a special boon in the middle of the night), and the hours that can be spent on family trips and excursions, because your built-in pure milk supply, always at the right temperature, and eminently at hand, gives you complete freedom of movement with your baby.

And have you ever realized the amount of money that is saved by eliminating formula, bottles, and so on? Viola Lennon once figured that six months' formula and baby food equaled the price of a major appliance, or cleaning help for that length of time.

Good Mothering

Breastfeeding is an integral part of good mothering. "Mothering" includes not only feeding the baby, but keeping him warm and comfortable, soothing his feelings of fear or anger, and letting him develop at his own pace. It means accepting him for what he is—a helpless baby, not a miniature adult. It means communicating to him through body and voice and giving him the opportunity to communicate back. It means babying the baby, and gently guiding the child. It means meeting his real needs gladly and fully at each age, without smothering him with attentions he doesn't want or need at that age. Here let us point out that a tiny baby's "wants" and "needs" are one and the same. He has an inexhaustible need to be loved for what he is—a person with his own individuality. Psychiatrists are showing us that the manner in which these early needs are met, or not met, often has a great deal to do with your baby's good or bad response to people and situations in later life. So the way you mother your child is important not only for you and for him, but for society as well.

No one can teach you good mothering; all we or anyone else can do is to direct you back to wise Nature's plan and to give you occasional suggestions. For instance, the very young baby likes the secure feeling of being snugly wrapped up and cuddled. At about three months, another need begins to emerge—he likes company from time to time, and you prop him up in the midst of the family now and again, instead of rushing to feed him or cuddle him when what he really wants is just to be sociable and to escape boredom. This is a perfectly true observation about most babies—but *your* three-month-old may be overstimulated and miserable if you impose it on him. You have to be sensitive to the individual needs of your own baby.

This sensitivity which helps you do the right thing at the right time, and which comes from knowing him, develops as you spend time with him, and it develops more quickly, and to a greater degree, if you are nursing your baby. The very closeness and intimacy of breastfeeding give you a quicker and surer perception of the feelings and needs of this tiny person, and how to meet them.

The deepest, truest spirit of mothering grows as you experience the quick, strong feeling of affection so natural between a nursing mother and her baby; as you develop a sure understanding of your baby's needs, and joy and confidence in your own ability to satisfy them; and as you see the happy dividends from this good relationship as the baby grows. It is a spirit first sensed, gradually understood, finally realized fully by the mother who nurses her baby.

Just as breastfeeding is not a *guarantee* of good mothering, so bottle feeding by no means necessarily rules it out. If you have tried unsuccessfully in the past to breastfeed, or if you thought that bottle feeding was the proper thing to do, you certainly need not feel guilty about having "bottled" these earlier babies. The most important thing is the love which you give your baby. But *now*, you will not want to settle for a substitute when you can have the real thing, nor to do things the hard, complicated way when there is a simple, beautiful, natural way. You'll see how much easier, better, more enjoyable it is to mother this baby you are planning to nurse.

Dividends for You

After you have brought your baby into the world, the first important step in your new role as a mother is putting your infant to your breast. The fact that you choose to take this step shows that you are already prepared to accept the obligations—and the joys—of motherhood. Having come this far on the road to maturity, you will find that the experience of giving yourself unstintingly to your child will bring you even further along. In other words, one of the ways in which breastfeeding will benefit *you* is by helping you become a more real, more loving person, in relation to others as well as to your child.

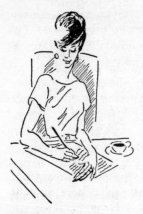

Mothers Write Us

We can assure you that this is not merely theorizing on our part. Time and again mothers talking to us or writing us have told of their personal experiences which, one way or another, serve to underscore the generalization we have just made. Let us quote for you from just three of the letters we have received:

> After three bottle-fed babies I am finally a successful nursing mother. The striking difference is the tremendous feeling of satisfaction that this baby has given *me*. Up till now I have been always completely baffled by the phrase "enjoy your baby." Not so with my breastfed baby. She, at three months, and I are already great friends. I feel as though I have finally arrived at motherhood. It's such a lovely warm glow that nursing imparts. And the nicest part of all is that this warm glow seems to be endless. It spills over into my relationships with all the rest of my family; there's always some to spare.—*Wilma S.*

> So much is written about nursing being best for baby; we know that. I think more should be written about what it does for the mother. Patti is our fifth child, the first to be breastfed. I am amazed at the difference in me. I had no idea what I was missing and I'm sure that if anyone even hinted at it I would have resented it. It is a feeling of growth and development—it is hard to describe, but I feel as if I have finally arrived (motherhood). I have such a sense of completeness, of fulfillment.—*Kay R.*

> After three babies who were not nursed and having a grandma readily available, I was free to come and go pretty much as I pleased. I was afraid that I might resent being tied down to my breastfed baby. On the contrary, however, being tied down is more than compensated for by this wonderful feeling of being needed. She needs me as no other person in the whole world ever has and no one else can take my place with her. On days when so many things have gone wrong and my own performance has not been creditable I get renewed and refreshed when I am nursing my baby and realize that with all my faults she loves me and needs me just the way I am. When I finally put her down I find I am calm again and kinder to the rest of the family.—*Gladys R.*

Added to these are the ever-growing observations made by the medical profession. Doctors have, of course, always attested to the benefits of breastfeeding. Now psychiatrists and psychologists are doing research on human emotions as they are related to care in infancy and early childhood. The importance of breastfeeding in this relationship has been stressed over and over again.

A Handful of Quotations

Breastfeeding is an art, and one much more worth studying than the far less dependable complexities of artificial feeding.—*Dr. Frank Howard Richardson*

Human milk should be considered superior to cow's milk as the initial physiologic food for the human infant. . . . Human milk is for the human infant, cow's milk is for the calf. . . . Breastfeeding reduces both morbidity and mortality rates, especially the latter.— *Dr. Paul Gyorgy*

A baby whose mother enjoys suckling him is less likely to develop eating difficulties later on.—*Dr. Melitta Schmideberg*

There is a special and intimate relationship between the milk of the mother and the needs of her own offspring.—*Dr. Truby King*

The newborn baby has only three demands. They are warmth in the arms of its mother, food from her breast, and security in the knowledge of her presence. Breastfeeding satisfies all three.—*Dr. Grantly Dick-Read*

Chapter 2

Planning for Baby

A CHANGE OF EMPHASIS

The first thing you will need to realize is that it just isn't possible to absorb a new baby into a rigid household schedule. Any routines you have set up for accomplishing your household tasks will certainly need revision. What is more, you will have to let go, not only the strict routines, but also the notion that, once the baby is older, you will get back to your original ways of doing things. You have to face the fact that this is not a temporary change, but an improvement in your way of living, just as marriage was both a change and an improvement. You now go one step further in your special vocation, motherhood.

We implied earlier, and we want to emphasize here, that raising a baby by charts and rules and schedules interferes with real mothering. Further, where any routine involved in running a house at top efficiency comes into conflict with the needs of one of the human beings sharing their lives in that house, it's the routine that has to give. Some girls who are perfect housekeepers may simply not have anything more important to do.

If you have older children, it's very likely that your own instincts led you to compromise with the schedule a good deal of the time when *they* were babies, so that they probably got a lot more mothering than a really rigid regime would have permitted. You'll be doing the same thing with this baby, and with a clear conscience.

The Rest of the Family

But, you ask, how about the needs of other members of the household? Won't the baby interfere with *them* sometimes?

He certainly will, and this is where the mutual love and understanding that cement good human relationships come in. You and your husband, and the older children if there are any, will talk about this from time to time during the months you are waiting for the new member of the family. Ask them to help you think of ways of managing that will be best for everyone, always remembering that the new baby will be the only member of the family who is completely dependent on you, so that his needs must certainly come first. Children understand this more readily than you might think. It is revealing, and gratifying, to us to find that a crying baby can be very disturbing to the older children. They sense that something is not right, and they are happy again only when baby is happy.

Still looking ahead, you'll find that cheerfully putting the needs of the baby first as a matter of course is really a fine thing for everyone concerned. It's truly a good way to educate your children for their future role as loving parents.

The older children will realize that they too came first when *they* were tiny, especially if you make a point of mentioning this from time to time, casually, before the baby comes. And after baby is here, there will be plenty of bits of dialogue: "Mary, when you were little and hungry, I'd tell Timmy and Elizabeth and the older ones to wait a bit because I wanted to feed *you*" (or rock you, or cuddle you, or whatever), in the tone of one sharing a happy reminiscence with someone who is still pretty special. Mary will love the idea of once having been the star.

So part of your planning will consist of enlisting the help of the rest of the family. They will probably come up

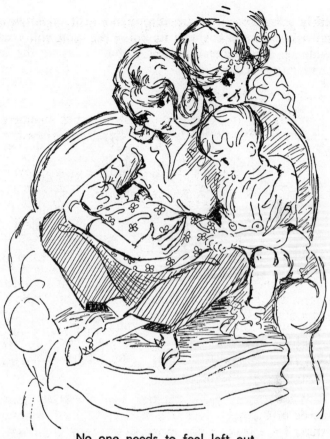

No one needs to feel left out

with some good suggestions if you ask them. We have a few suggestions for you too, mostly on ways of simplifying your life after the baby comes.

Meal Planning

If your family has been used to home-baked goodies every night, as one of their contributions to the new member of the family they can graciously settle for fresh fruit. It's better for them anyhow, nutritionally speaking. You can work out a few ultra-simple menus now and stock your shelves accordingly. Then on the days when baby is awake when he's "supposed" to be asleep, and your meal preparations have to be cut to just a few minutes, you will be able to whip up a good meal quickly without denying the baby your much-needed attention.

Cleaning and Laundry

If this is your first baby, the house isn't going to need much in the way of cleaning. Again, if you have older children, let them help all they are able—but beware of overdoing this. Don't expect too much of them, and do be quick to let them know that you appreciate their help and unselfishness. Also beware of making a practice of going all out for cleaning, cooking, scrubbing, and so on, whenever the baby is taking a nap. Give some of that time to the other children. They don't need you as much as the baby does, but they too are more important than the house.

Laundry, of course, is more urgent than cleaning house. Sometimes you may be able to send some of it out or have someone in to help with it. If not, you'll probably find yourself washing smaller loads several days a week and perhaps ironing for just fifteen minutes a day instead of trying to get it all done at once.

Easy Does It

In other words, with parenthood, your goal becomes clearer. It isn't any longer so important to you to keep a spotless house. It and its furnishings will be around a long time; but you will never get back your child's babyhood or childhood. So let the chores wait and keep your family happy, no matter how much time this may demand.

As for help—accept thankfully all offers to take over your housework, cooking, or laundry chores for a time, but remember that no one can be as good a mother to your baby as you can. Beware of offers to "relieve you of the baby." There will be plenty of time to share your child with Grandma when he is no longer a dependent infant. In the early weeks, if you get fatigued, you'll just take the baby with you and climb into bed. And if Grandma or anyone else wants to work around the house and get a meal on the table while you and the baby sleep—God bless them.

When it comes to getting husband and older children off to work or school on time, you may have to use a little ingenuity. Betty Wagner, mother of seven, manages by setting the alarm for about twenty minutes earlier than her regular get-up time. When it wakes her, she resets the alarm for the regular time, takes the baby up, and gets back into bed to nurse him. Then when she does have to get breakfast and do other rush things, at least she knows the baby isn't hungry. There's where some of that family type teamwork comes in handy, too. Children love working alongside mother. Breakfast can become a group operation. (Keep it up, too, when the baby is older. It's a fine way for children to learn a bit about cooking and so on.)

In general, just resign yourself to living a more easygoing kind of life. Pretty soon you will find you like it that way. So will your friends. "Keeping up with the Joneses" can be awfully wearing for everyone. Lots of mothers would be only too glad to know that you don't care if the breakfast dishes aren't done before lunch. They'll follow suit and we'll all relax.

YOU PLAN AHEAD

Your Husband Helps Plan

Your husband will want to be in on your planning before the baby comes. You may or may not have to convince him that breastfeeding is right for his child. Most husbands are enthusiastic about the idea from the start; they know without much thinking about it that it is not only the best way but the *womanly* way to feed a baby; and womanliness is the trait they most value in a wife. So you will probably be able to lean heavily on your husband for moral support and encouragement. You may need to if other relatives and friends don't go along with the idea. In any case, keep him informed about what you learn about breastfeeding and how you feel about it. Plans made by the two of you together will usually work out better than any you might make by yourself. (The whole subject of the father's role is discussed more fully in Chapter 8.)

Your Doctor Is In on It

As for the doctor you choose, we suggest that you tell him at your first prenatal visit that you want to breastfeed this baby. Different doctors will react differently to this announcement, so from here on you will more or less have to play it by ear. If he is enthusiastic and knowledgeable about breastfeeding, fine. If he approves in a theoretical sort of way, but hasn't had occasion to concentrate on the practical aspects of breastfeeding, you can reassure him that you have a *wonderful* book by some experienced mothers, who have even invited you to write or phone them about any practical problems that might come up. In a few cases, he may throw cold water on the whole idea. If that happens, don't let your confidence in yourself be shaken. We know many women who have successfully nursed their babies and enjoyed it thoroughly even though their doctors haven't been able to understand "why they wanted to bother." If the doctor feels very negative about it, try to find out why. In this case you definitely need to be in touch with some mother who knows the ins and outs of breastfeeding because of her own successful personal experience. If you don't know one, by all means get in touch with us (see the section "About La Leche League" at the end of this book).

Of course, it will be better all around if your doctor does approve of breastfeeding, and this is one of the things to keep in mind when you choose him. Remember, your right and privilege as a patient is the choice of a doctor sympathetic to your needs and desires. (The American Medical Association calls this the Fifth Freedom.)

You'll want to talk with your doctor, too, about what to expect in the hospital you'll be going to. Is it geared to the needs of nursing mothers? If so, fine. If not, you and your doctor may need to plan your strategy ahead of time. He knows the hospital, and he'll be able to advise you on the best tactics. Also, there are several things he can do about the hospital situation that you can't (see pages 53-54). But remember that he's a busy man, and if most of his maternity patients don't nurse their babies, some of these details may slip his mind unless you remind him when you get to the hospital. Make a mental note now to do this.

You Learn about Childbirth

Another subject you will be discussing with your doctor early in pregnancy is your delivery. He will explain to you how all the forces operating within you at that time are directed toward the birth of your baby, and how your voluntary physical participation supports and assists in this.

An appreciation of how thoroughly your body is preparing itself for what takes place during labor and delivery has great value. To learn more about normal childbirth you can read some of the many books published on this subject (see Booklist, page 141). You might also ask if classes in childbirth education are available in your area. If you can't find out locally, contact the International Childbirth Education Association (ICEA), Box 5852, Milwaukee, Wisconsin 53220; or the American Society for Psycho-Prophylaxis in Obstetrics (ASPO), 7 West 96 Street, New York, N.Y. 10025.

In these classes you learn with other expectant mothers what will happen during labor and delivery. You learn how to relax through a series of breathing techniques and simple exercises. You learn that the use of these techniques lessens the need for drugs or medications, often to the point where none is needed. (Doctors, too, are happier when the desire for drugs is lessened or eliminated.) You learn that relaxing your body permits the spontaneous forces of labor to perform their functions more effectively, making the delivery of your baby smoother, safer, and shorter. When you understand what is happening to you and your developing infant from now until he is born, any fears, doubts and misconceptions will take flight. Soon you begin to look forward each day with greater anticipation to the birth of your child.

During childbirth, the emphasis is placed from the very beginning on the accomplishments of you, the mother. You are the central figure, but you are not alone. Your physician will be there, prepared to give you all the help you need: to encourage you if encouragement is needed and to assist you with his special skills.

By delivering your baby through alert participation and active cooperation, you are given the opportunity to achieve a rich, joyful, and maturing experience which will go a long way toward moving you to fuller womanhood and motherhood. We who have experienced this can only say that the joy of delivering your own baby and hearing his first cry will mark the crowning moment of achievement in your life. The second step of mothering your newborn, breastfeeding, flows from this as day follows night. Your love goes out immediately toward your child and moves you to take him to your breast at once. There is no blank gap between the start of labor and the holding of your new baby in your arms for the first time. This outflow of love and warmth for your child at this time—bewildered as he may be by his ejection from the womb—is an orderly continuation of the comfort, security, and warmth he has known for so long before his birth. Thus, your lifelong relationship with your child begins immediately upon his birth, and his first contact with the world is a soothing and satisfying one for both of you. This is what encourages your milk to come in sooner and speeds your way to successful nursing.

Furthermore, the loving encouragement your husband can give you during your labor is most important to your success as a mother. His presence is a source of strength to you and a great comfort. Your satisfaction in accomplishing this labor of love is more meaningful when reflected in his eyes. For the father, this experience binds him to his child, and to the mother of his child, in a very special way.

Childbirth, then, can be—and should be—a rich family experience, shared by husband and wife, as they join together to greet this new gift from God, their baby. It is a wonderful beginning for baby, mother, and father.

With all this clear in your mind, you can settle down to wait for the arrival of your baby.

Do Some More Reading

Especially if this is your first baby, you will have the time and the inclination to do a lot of reading about babies. This is a good thing. You may be expecting a baby shower or a few gifts from cheering friends and relatives. If so, you can let it be known that you would like a book or two from the list on pages 141-146, and hope that some one will take the hint. Or you can exchange such items as beautiful, gleaming sterilizers and fancy little bottle warmers for some of the books. In a pinch, you can always buy them yourself, or borrow them. Most of them can be obtained at the public library. One thing to guard against in many books is that the advice is often based on the assumption that your baby will be bottle fed. Learn to detect and ignore those parts.

What to Wear

You will be glad to shed your maternity garb when your figure changes to the smaller tummy and temporarily fuller bust of the nursing mother. Actually, you can make almost any clothes do for nursing, but we have a few suggestions that can make it easier for an active mother. You might as well be getting them ready.

Most mothers find nursing bras very practical. You can use at least two or three. In deciding on the number of bras you want, bear in mind that you may find it more comfortable to wear one in bed for a while. The kind of bra with a little "trap door" is good, especially if it is a combination maternity and nursing bra which you can wear both during pregnancy and for nursing. Avoid anything that takes a lot of fumbling and fussing to manage, or bras that are too tight. They may flatten the nipples or press on the milk ducts. If the bra has a plastic liner, be sure it doesn't touch the skin. Either remove it or insert padding. (You might try your husband's clean hanky folded to fit.)

Half-slips are probably handiest, but if they leave you cold around the midriff in wintry weather, you can adapt full slips to your needs. Loosen the straps in the front from the adjustment clips, and when you dress in the morning, fasten them to your bra straps with small safety pins or paper clips, which you leave in the rest of the day. Tuck the top of the bodice into the top of your bra to keep it in place, or use snaps or hooks and eyes if you prefer. At feeding time, simply drop the bodice portion.

For outer apparel, two-piece outfits—skirts or slacks or shorts plus blouses or sweaters—are simple around the house and especially good for nursing when you're away from home. You'll find that they permit you to nurse so unobtrusively that even someone sitting next to you won't know what you are doing. Pulled up just enough, a sweater, knit top, or blouse (with bottom buttons opened) won't look any different above, and baby covers any bare midriff.

Those one-piece dresses with back or side openings don't have to gather dust in the closet if you are handy with a needle and thread. Many of them can easily be adapted to unobtrusive nursing. Most of them have a dart on each side of the front running from waist to bust; some of them may have a seam there. You simply rip the seam, cutting the dart open if necessary, then bind each side with a wide strip of seam binding—or of the same material if you prefer and can sneak some from a hem or some place else. Sew the opening again, leaving four inches or so to be fastened by snaps (two or more, depending on the weight of the material) or a zipper.

Dresses that open down the front are easy, and you can look as sharp as the next one. They are harder to manage, though, as far as inconspicuous nursing goes.

Baby Furniture

There are so many kinds of special furniture and gadgets for baby that you can indulge your inclinations just as far as your own pocketbook and the generosity of the cheering section permit. There are four items, though, that we'd like to recommend. Bear in mind that these are nice, though not absolutely necessary.

First, a comfortable rocking chair, with or without a footstool, as you prefer. You'll find this worth its weight in gold during the later stages of your pregnancy, especially if you are at home during the early stages of labor. After the baby is born, we all consider it perhaps the most indispensable piece of furniture we own.

Second, a basket, cradle, buggy or some other kind of babytoter that can be carried easily or wheeled around the house with you. This is in addition to the full-size crib that stays put in the bedroom. Incidentally, you can get a fine bouncy rocking motion to that full-size crib by replacing the wheels with special springs designed for this purpose.

Third, a car bed that can be put on the floor behind the front seat (the *safest* spot). This could double as the babytoter for indoors, too, if you like.

Fourth, some kind of canvas sling for toting baby when you are on foot. There is one kind that holds him astride

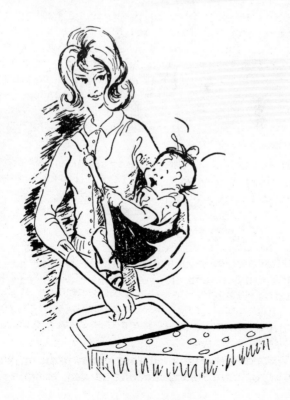

your hip. The one we prefer for shopping, hiking, bike riding, ironing, or what have you, goes on the back like a knapsack, with holes for the legs to go through, and is big

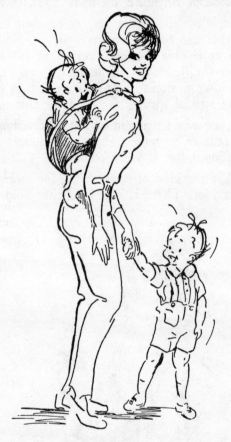

enough to allow a comfortable fit over diapers and snow suits. However, this kind can't usually be put into service until the baby is four or five months old and can hold his head up fairly well.

Your Diet

We take it for granted that you will be making sure you are getting an adequate diet during pregnancy. (See the next chapter if you aren't sure what an adequate diet consists of.) Follow whatever special suggestions your doctor gives you. Then continue these good eating habits while you are nursing baby and make them standard household fare from then on.

To Smoke or Not to Smoke

Smoking, either while you are carrying the baby or while you are nursing him, does him no good; but if you are a smoker, the problem of eliminating this habit may be too much for you. If you *would* like to stop, your pregnancy may make it easier for you to do so by giving you an additional motive. Studies have indicated that there may be a connection between heavy smoking and prematurity or miscarriages. We'd suggest stopping if you want to and can; otherwise, do try to cut down a bit, during pregnancy rather than later, since more nicotine gets through to the baby while you are carrying him than later through the milk.

Drugs During Pregnancy

One rule our medical advisors insist on is: don't take *any* medication whatsoever unless it is definitely necessary and has been prescribed or approved by your own physician. This rule applies throughout life and for all members of your family, but it is particularly applicable during the first half of pregnancy—a fact sharply underlined by the thalidomide tragedies. Dr. Helen B. Taussig of Johns Hopkins University writes: "Young women must learn that nothing is foolproof and new drugs should not be taken unless absolutely necessary, as the damage often occurs before the woman knows she is pregnant."

So follow the rule: *no* medication unless prescribed or approved by your physician. It is *imperative* for you to follow this rule during your pregnancy; it's *advisable* for you to share this good health practice with your husband and the children. We live in an age of overmedication and an increasingly high incidence of serious drug allergies and other sometimes tragic reactions. Strict following of the simple rule above will help protect your family's health—and, incidentally, will have a noticeably beneficial effect on the family budget.

PRENATAL NIPPLE CARE

You may or may not run into any difficulty with your nipples if you give them no special care during pregnancy. Many women who don't bother with any special preparations beforehand never have any trouble with sore nipples, no matter how long or how often their baby nurses. However, some women, especially redheads and others with fair complexions, do have difficulty with tenderness or soreness; and since you can't tell ahead of time, it is wise to follow a few simple preparatory routines.

Your regular bath is all the washing the nipples will require, now or later. Go easy on the soap. Many of us eliminate soap entirely for a while in bathing the nipple area. If you must use it, do so sparingly and rinse well, because soap is drying to the skin and dryness encourages cracked nipples.

Hand-Expression

It is sometimes recommended that you hand-express a few drops of colostrum from each breast every day during the last six weeks of pregnancy, and you may want to do this, with your doctor's approval. Colostrum is the fluid secreted before the milk comes in, which doctors say is so important for the newborn baby and one good reason (there are others) why you should nurse your baby as soon after delivery as possible. The reason for expressing the colostrum daily for a few weeks before the baby is born is to open the milk ducts, thereby reducing the engorgement which sometimes occurs when the milk first comes in and which some mothers find quite uncomfortable.

Hand-expression is quite simple. It is the same whether you are expressing colostrum during pregnancy or milk later on. Wash your hands. Cup the breast in your hand, placing your thumb above and forefinger below the breast at the edge of the dark area (areola), and simply squeeze thumb and finger together, gently. Don't slide the finger and thumb out toward the nipple. Don't worry if nothing comes out the first few times you try it. You'll get the knack soon. Rotate your hand slightly back and forth several times in order to reach all the milk ducts, which radiate out from the nipple.

A Daily Routine

Although some women are never bothered with sore nipples no matter how long or how often their babies nurse, others occasionally have some trouble. Many women have found it helpful to do the following exercise once or twice daily to condition the nipples. Pull out the nipple several times quite firmly—only until it is slightly uncomfortable, never painful. It's a good idea to use an oily lubricant during this daily treatment. Pure lanolin is fine; cold cream or baby oil will do nicely.

Expressing the colostrum and pulling out the nipples take only a few minutes. You can work them into your daily routine quite comfortably. When you are dressing or undressing is a good time. The important thing is to be regular about it during the last several weeks of pregnancy.

The obstetrician who first recommended this procedure to us claims that any mother who follows it faithfully will not have sore or cracked nipples—they may be tender for a while, but never worse. Our experience and that of many mothers to whom we have suggested this kind of nipple care tend to confirm this.

Inverted Nipples

If you have flat or inverted nipples, you may not be able to carry out the recommended nipple care as easily as the mother with protruding nipples; but work at it and eventually you will find you can manage. A little practice now will save a lot of time and maybe some mental anguish after the baby is born. One mother who has this kind of nipple has called it "the folding model of the nipple world"; there is a real full-sized nipple there, ready and able to do the job for which it was intended, but it folds back into the breast when not in use. Completely inverted nipples are quite rare, and they can be a nuisance. On the other hand, rather flat, even depressed nipples, which are quite common, respond to the kind of treatment suggested above. You may not be able to decide which kind you have. If you suspect that you may have inverted nipples, watch them when you are expressing the colostrum. If they react to the squeezing pressure of your thumb and finger by coming out, even a little, this is not a true inverted nipple. Even though you may not be able to get it out very far now, the baby will later on.

If the nipples react to the pressure of hand-expression by retreating (exceptional, but it sometimes happens), then you do have inverted nipples; and you will have to work a little harder at getting them in condition for nursing, because you won't be able to get hold of them to pull. The thing is, you *have* to get them out some for the baby to be able to latch on. Once he can take hold, he will carry on from there.

The best treatment for bringing out truly inverted nipples is the use of Woolwich breast shields,* worn during pregnancy before the baby is born. Sometimes a mother may discover after the baby is born that she has an inverted nipple she never suspected; or, more often, her nipples may be temporarily retracted because of engorgement. The Woolwich shields may be useful at this time too, worn between feedings. If it's simply engorgement, just the time between two feedings may do the trick. In more severe cases it may be necessary to wear them for a day or two or even for two or three weeks. The mother should not save the milk that leaks into the shields to feed the baby, and she is advised to wash the shields frequently with hot soapy water, rinse thoroughly, and dry carefully. She should try to leave the nipples exposed to the air for fifteen to thirty minutes several times each day.

---

* These have been used successfully by English obstetricians for over thirty years. If you can't obtain them locally, they are available from La Leche League for $3.75 a pair (plus postage). Complete, simple directions come with them.

Chapter 3

Nutritional Know-How For Nursing Mothers

The title of this chapter might be a little misleading, because it could be thought to imply that nursing mothers need a special diet. This is not true. If you already have good eating habits, there is no reason for you to make any major changes now. On the other hand, if you know that your eating habits could stand improvement, the period while you are pregnant and then nursing your baby is a good time to do this. You now have a strong motive in your baby's welfare as well as your own—and changes made because of strong motivation are easier to make and more likely to stick.

Your baby will get off to a fine start on your milk, a nutritionally perfect food for the infant. You will want him to build on this good start so that when he grows up he will have good eating habits. The best way to accomplish this is by being a family in which *everyone* has good nutritional habits. These then can become the baby's, as he grows, by imitation. Therefore, start improving your habits, if you feel they need improvement, while you are expecting this baby. By the time he is admitted to the family table, these habits will be taken as a matter of course by everyone.

With this goal in mind, we would like to give you some

general principles of food selection and utilization. We think broad understanding of how Nature relates to you nutritionally is most important. We believe this understanding to be more valuable than chemical analyses or detailed food lists as a guide in choosing the foods you and your family need for good health. It is also simpler.

Because we have nowhere found this sensible approach better stated than by Dr. Herbert Ratner,* we have followed his remarks almost verbatim in the paragraphs that follow. Then, having equipped you with a basic understanding of the principles of good nutrition, we will add a few practical suggestions that come out of our experiences with our own families, as well as some special hints for nursing mothers.

THE BASIC APPROACH

Knowing about foods and what foods are good for you is really a simple matter. Although it is valuable to have as much knowledge about foods as possible, you don't have to be a physician, or a chemist, or a nutritionist, or a dietician, to eat well. You don't have to know what vitamins, and minerals, and proteins are to feed yourself well. Human beings successfully survived innumerable centuries before the sciences and scientists existed. So for our purposes here, to make this practical, let's try to forget about science and technical words and try to get the whole problem of nutrition simplified.

First, however, it should be made clear that in special disease situations, scientific knowledge of foods can help you to choose the foods your special needs demand; but these *are* special situations. When needed, such a dietary can and should be worked out with your individual physician. What we're discussing, however, is a practical approach to nutrition for the well person, not the sick person.

The first thing you have to appreciate is what a wonder-

---

*In a short monograph prepared and distributed by the Oak Park (Ill.) Health Department, which was adapted from a talk presented on a television program entitled *Nutrition and Public Health,* one of a series of thirteen kinescopes prepared for educational television use by ONSET, the Organization for the National Support of Educational Television, 1958.

ful mechanism the human appetite is. It's geared to health. It's the most sensitive biological mechanism that exists. Respect it. Your appetite leads you to grow well, to develop properly, and, as an adult, to maintain the exact same weight year after year—barring, of course, whatever bad habits you may have developed.

The appetite—if it isn't seduced (by delicacies), or confused (by sweets), or misdirected (by emotional hungers)—will see to it that you don't eat too little, that you don't eat too much, and that you eat the kinds of foods you need. In the presence of natural foods, the appetite is virtually foolproof. In man, as in all other animals, if the opportunity for a natural selection is there, the appetite will always direct itself and demand the right foods at the right times. And herein lies the secret of good nutrition: proper food selection.

Here the cardinal principle is that Nature is the best manufacturer and supplier of man's dietary needs. This should be understood in a twofold way. First, that the living animals and plants upon which our nutrition depends are the best source of all those food elements needed for optimum life, as proven by their own capacity to thrive. Second, that these sources of food, generally speaking, contain all our chemical needs (minerals, vitamins, acids, alkalies, etc.) in proper balance and proportions.

How, then, do you go about selecting food, in addition to the overall guide of digestibility?

Eat a Variety of Foods

First, you should eat a variety of animals and plants. You shouldn't concentrate on one animal like the cow, or other such four-legged animals, to the exclusion of feathered animals, like fowl; or land animals to the exclusion of water animals like fish or sea food. In the plant kingdom, you shouldn't restrict yourself to certain vegetables, to the exclusion of fruit, nuts, grains, and cereals; green vegetables to the exclusion of orange vegetables; the bland to the exclusion of the sweet or tart.

Women instinctively seek a diversity of clothes and

colors to decorate their bodies. The *inner* body also has needs. That is why women, who have the great gift of diversification and are the cooks, should seek a diversity of textures and colors for their tables. The body thrives on a diversity of foods and a diversity of flavors, colors, even textures—chewy, soft, firm, juicy, crisp. All of the different textures, colors, and flavors of food reflect different food elements and values needed for the body, as clothes, in their way, manifest the varying elements in a woman's personality and vocation. In each case, variety supplies a true need: for the woman, a psychological need; for the body, a physiological or nutritional need. And these are not unrelated, for we have been given the highest combination of sense organs and perceptions for a reason: to be able to take in the world, both figuratively and literally.

Secondly, you should eat a variety of the parts of animals and plants, the parts that make up the whole. We want to have whole health, not just partial health. In animals, you shouldn't just concentrate on muscle (for the most part the expensive cuts), such as steaks, chops, roasts. There are also liver, tongue, sweetbreads, hearts, kidneys, gizzards, spareribs, even soup bones. And there's also the old-fashioned catchall, farm sausage. There are milk, cheese, and eggs.

In plants—the parts don't have to belong to the same plant—there are leaves, like the greens that go into a salad, as well as spinach and cabbage. There are roots, like carrots, beets, yams, turnips, and radishes. There are stems and tubers, like asparagus and potatoes, and the fruits of the plant, like corn, string beans, and tomatoes, as well as apples, oranges, grapes, bananas, and melons.

There is even variety obtainable in fats, which are so important to the cooking and preparation of foods and which also compactly supply large amounts of energy. In these uncertain scientific times, reflected in fancy scientific adjectives featured in food advertising, it is refreshing to know that there is a simpler approach to good fat nutrition. There are animal fats and vegetable fats. There are solid fats and liquid fats. Of the animal fats there are butter, cream, lard, and chicken fat. There are vegetable oils such as olive, corn,

cottonseed, and peanut. There are even fish oils. We all
know of the important role cod-liver oil has played in the
history of man. By extending our food preparation habits
from the animal fats to the broader use of the many vegetable
oils available to us, we don't have to bother our heads with
such terms as polysaturated and polyunsaturated, or essential
and nonessential fatty acids.

Eat Natural Foods

By eating natural foods, you can—and should—respect
your likes and dislikes as long as your dislikes don't exclude
so many things that you end up eating few types of food,
or as long as you do not impose your dislikes on the rest of
the family. After all, you don't want your children to grow
up with crippled eating habits. Furthermore, your dislikes
should never lead you to exclude any of the four basic groups:
the milk, meat, vegetable and fruit, and bread and cereal
groups.

If there is a particular food you or other members of
your family dislike, there is always a substitute. Cheese is a
good substitute for milk. Eggs are a good substitute for meat
and fish. Dried peas and beans, and nuts, are good occasional
substitutes and supplements for meats. This is the lovely
thing about Nature. She provides such a variety of foods
that every culture in every age, whether in Europe, or Asia or
elsewhere, has had a varied selection available to it. It has resulted, among other things, in a wondrous variety of national
dishes: French, Chinese, Italian, Hawaiian, German, Japanese,
Austrian, Polish, Spanish. In the United States today, the
selection available to you is especially wide. First, because
modern transportation and mechanization make possible a
varied and diverse selection of foods all through the year
by sharing the productive seasons and rich bounty of other
parts of the country and the world with you. Secondly,
because America is the great melting pot of the world. The
Irish eat pizza, the Italians eat hot pastrami on rye, business-
men eat chop suey, teenagers eat African lobster tails. Shopping in a contemporary supermarket gets to be more and
more like taking a tour around the nation and the world.

So you don't all have to eat a uniform diet; you can eat what you want in terms of the culture you're accustomed to, or the new cultures you explore. For, as one mother used to say, philosophizing about her daughter-in-law's strange cooking, which she reluctantly enjoyed, "If you put good things into it, why shouldn't it come out tasting good?" There are many, many different ways of achieving good nutrition without eating the same foods.

One other point should be made here. Generally speaking, the further one gets away from the natural state, the poorer the food nutritionally. From this point of view, many foods are better raw than cooked. This has special applicability to fruits and vegetables. Undercooked foods, with due allowance for digestibility, are better than overcooked foods. Here we can learn much from the Chinese. Frozen foods, generally speaking, are better than canned. Lastly, the fewer the food additives the better.

The advantages that will accrue from this kind of an approach to the diet should be obvious. By partaking of all the digestible parts of the living whole, and by concentrating on natural foods, you will get all of the known nutrient essentials in proper and natural proportions rather than in artificial concentrates: knife and fork and hand nutrients rather than pills. You will get all of the essential nutrients which have been discovered by science, and those which have yet to be discovered; not only the vitamins and minerals of today, but the vitamins and minerals of tomorrow. This approach is also more economical, and it doesn't require a science course. To top it all off, it will protect you against ill health and at the same time supply you with a variety of choices to make everyone happy.

What to Avoid

There's one major danger that must be emphasized. Civilization, although it has brought much progress, has also introduced some evils which have created a real problem in nutrition. The appetite, man's inherent guide to good nutrition, has been confused by highly refined and unnatural foods—two products of modern food technology. Because the appetite has been thus confused, poor tastes and poor food habits have developed, and, in many instances, poor nutrition has resulted.

The chief offender is sugar. It is the principal confuser and seducer of the appetite. We are thinking, here, of sugar in the form of rich desserts, pastries, cakes, candies, and soft drinks. A highly refined food like sugar can be easily misused and is bad, primarily, because it satisfies hunger needs and displaces the healthful, natural foods, especially in the young. Sugar in the form of natural foods, of course, such as fruit, is always all right, but in an artificial and concentrated form it should be used sparingly and saved for special, festive occasions. Fluoridation notwithstanding, we will always have dental caries with us wherever the intake of refined sugar is high.

A second offender is highly processed cereals and grains which have been converted, in processing, from natural to unnatural foods. These processed cereals and grains rob us of important minerals and vitamins. What we have to do is reacquire a taste for products made out of whole grain: whole-wheat flour, cracked wheat, rolled oats, graham flour, unpolished rice, and whole-grain ready-to-eat breakfast cereals.

You may know that to correct this latter problem the *enrichment process* was developed—a process, in this instance, designed to replace what was lost in processing. From the public health point of view, this was the most efficient way to handle the nutritional deficiencies that were occurring because of our preference in this country for refined foods —white instead of yellow or brown, fine instead of coarse. Furthermore, public health had to contend with the problem of improving suboptimal diets due to the poorer economic status of earlier decades and their lower food budgets, and again the enrichment process was the most efficient way. You must remember, however, that this enrichment is only an enrichment of an inferior product, not of a superior product. It is only an imitation of the original. It is only an attempt by man to make the unnatural simulate the natural through scientific and technological skill, which is always dated. Therefore, it must not be forgotten that the imitation only approximates the perfection of the normal or natural. The original always remains preferred. Today, our improved economic status, plus the talents and economies of modern food merchandizing, has changed the picture considerably. Superior nutrition through a wiser selection and greater availability of natural foods has never been more possible.

If you follow the basic principles we have outlined—and add the womanly art of making foods tasty and attractive and of serving foods with love—you and your family will never suffer nutritionally. The body is the wisest manufacturing plant that was ever made or created. All it asks is that you wisely choose for it a proper and diverse selection of natural foods daily.

PRACTICAL SUGGESTIONS

If your family has been used to eating only muscle meats, white bread, and a few vegetables, don't expect them to change their food habits overnight. Introducing new foods requires tact, patience, and imagination. Here are some suggestions that have worked for us:

1. Try serving small pieces of liver on the same platter with lots of bacon. Cook the bacon first, then quickly cook the liver in the hot bacon drippings, so that the smell of the bacon is in the air. If you like onions, slice some on top of the liver as it browns. Then when the liver "fingers" are brown on both sides, add a little water, stirring just a bit so the liver doesn't stick, cover, and let simmer for a few minutes.

2. Ask the butcher to grind a beef heart like hamburger. Start out by mixing half heart and half hamburger (half-heartedly, you might say) and use in meatloaf, spaghetti, chili, barbecue dishes, or just as hamburgers. Later you might want to use the ground heart alone. This dish is kind on your food budget. There are many other appetizing ways of serving variety and low-cost meats.

3. Liquid fats such as corn oil can be worked into the diet in homemade salad dressings, pies, bread, and pancakes.

Such a change would be good if you have been using mostly animal fats.

4. A simple way to introduce whole-grain products to your family is by baking your own bread. Start out by adding small amounts of whole-wheat flour to the white and gradually increase the amount over a period of months until the 100% whole-wheat loaf is no longer strange tasting and even becomes more desirable than the insipid white loaf. Very young children whose tastes have not had time to become conditioned usually like it right away. It is tasty! Older children can be given "half and half" sandwiches for awhile—one half whole-wheat, the other half white bread.

5. Your family may also take to the addition of wheat germ in their diet. Wheat germ can be bought at most grocery stores, is very tasty, and can be used in diverse ways. It can be added to any ground meat mixture, peanut butter, and most bread, cookie, pancake, and waffle mixtures. It can also be sprinkled on top of cereals. Labels that come on the wheat germ container usually carry a variety of good recipes.

6. Acquire the habit of reading the labels on food packages. In looking for whole-wheat bread, for example, if the label reads "wheat flour" it refers to the usual white flour. It must say "whole wheat" to mean that. You can avoid many unnecessary fillers and sugar by reading and comparing labels.

7. Make between-meal snacks nutritious and not just something to fill up on. Fresh fruit, dried fruit, nuts, carrot and celery sticks are fine. If the children are starving and supper isn't ready, pass around a tray of salad fixings (without the dressing), or glasses of fruit or vegetable juice; or hand out pieces of raw vegetables as you prepare them for the meal. Many's the nutritious morsel that has been gobbled avidly when handed out rather reluctantly beforehand that might have been scorned when it appeared, cooked and decorous, on a dinner plate. This reminds us of a mother of ten children who routinely cooks only half of the vegetables for a meal, serving the remainder raw at the table so each child can take his choice.

SOME SPECIAL HINTS FOR NURSING MOTHERS

We remarked earlier that if you have good eating habits, there is no reason for you to make any major changes when you are carrying or nursing a baby. You do have to remember to eat enough to keep yourself in good shape—eating well is part of being a good mother. It isn't the baby, either before or after birth, that will suffer markedly from your poor eating habits. The baby gets preferential treatment through breast milk in respect to his nutritional needs. Your body, with the deep wisdom of Nature, keeps right on making the right kind of milk to the best of its ability given the materials at hand. However, the baby, as well as the rest of the family, will suffer if the mother is tired and dragged out from skipping breakfast or taking "a bite on the run" for lunch.

Many mothers have reported the good result they get from taking brewer's yeast, which is Nature's vitamin-B complex concentrate. Some feel that it definitely helps increase their milk supply; others report that it is a remarkable help in combatting fatigue, depression, and irritability. Of course, the best way to combat these bugbears of motherhood is by improving your daily diet and getting enough rest; but if you feel you need extra help, brewer's yeast might be just that for you. It is a natural food containing not only the B-complex vitamins (often called the nerve vitamins) but also large amounts of iron and protein. Although the powdered yeast can be bitter, some stores have a palatable powder which mixes easily in juice or milk. Many find this more convenient than taking a number of tablets daily.

A Few Reminders

Nursing mothers just naturally feel the need for extra liquids. A nursing mother needs plenty of water—either "straight" or in the form of fruit and vegetable juices, milk, soup, or what-have-you—and in the excitement and bustle of a new baby, you may not always notice that you are dry and thirsty. Some mothers take a drink of water just before each nursing. If your urine is not concentrated (darker in color and small in amount), you are probably drinking all you need. Constipation may be a secondary sign of inadequate fluids. If you get constipated, increase your liquid intake, especially fruit juices. Avoid fancy remedies. Several mothers have told us that they get in a good supply of prune juice and prunes in their last month of pregnancy and continue with this from the day they come home. They find it easier thus to avoid rather than to cure the constipation which sometimes follows childbirth.

If you don't like milk, don't force yourself to drink it. Rather, to compensate, increase your intake of other dairy products and perhaps add nonfat dry milk to foods you do enjoy. Coffee and tea are all right in moderation. If you are getting at least half your liquids in water, juice, and milk, and the rest in coffee and tea, then you can consider this a moderate amount. Remember that soft drinks contain lots of sugar and little or no food value and are a bad and expensive example for your children.

We'd better repeat here what we said about smoking during pregnancy, since the same principle applies while you are nursing. It does the baby no good, and if you can quit without much difficulty, by all means do so. Many smokers don't believe they can. Then do the next best thing —cut down some if you can, and don't worry about it. It's more important for the baby to have a relaxed, happy mother than a nonsmoking one, if he can't have both.

Supplements

We do not take, and we would not advise you to take, any vitamin or mineral preparations except those specifically prescribed by the doctor. They are more expensive and not as much fun as good food. You may actually do yourself more harm than good by taking too much of them, or by taking them in unbalanced amounts.

Your doctor may advise supplementary vitamins and minerals for you during pregnancy, particularly iron, to replenish and build up your stores from which your baby is building up his own supply of iron to carry him through his first half-year of life.

During the nursing period, your doctor, rather than

prescribing vitamins and minerals directly to the baby, may prefer you to take them, to make certain that you are on an optimum nutritional diet.

We like to exchange good nutritious recipes, and a while back we printed a collection of these in a book we call MOTHER'S IN THE KITCHEN (see page 145).

A Word About Dieting

If you are overweight after your baby arrives, by more than about ten pounds, a little extra effort to take off the excess will do no harm either to you or to your baby, provided you're sensible about it. Don't go on a crash diet or a lopsided one. Stick to the basic foods, only decrease the portions somewhat, especially where sweets, starches, and fats are concerned. Losing a pound a week is a good goal to strive for and should be easily attained without interfering with your switch to better permanent eating habits. Breastfeeding your baby need never be an excuse for overweight.

It must be remembered, however, that some additional poundage accumulated during pregnancy is frequently Nature's intent. Pregnancy is a kind of hibernating period that prepares you for the extra energies that go into getting an infant through his first year. Moderately extra weight in the form of stored fat is protective. It comes in quite handy, given the additional energy requirements associated with the increased activity of caring for a bouncing baby and with the increased exercise that comes from handling a newborn who triples his weight by the end of the year. This increased activity (plus nursing, which helps burn extra calories) is Nature's postnatal body conditioner and physical fitness routine. If by the end of the year you are not back to your original streamlined self, you can check your eating habits. An honest appraisal and a little common sense will soon restore that svelte figure, and you'll be in tiptop condition physiologically too, because as a nursing mother you have been completely feminine, completely in harmony with the wonderful natural functioning of your body.

Chapter 4

Some Common Worries and Old Wives' Tales

In this chapter we are going to comment on some of the more common worries and misconceptions which you may have heard about breastfeeding. Every so often one of the mothers we talk with or correspond with comes up with a new one. But we believe you will find most of them included here, along with the truth of the matter.

What if My Breasts Aren't Adapted to Breastfeeding?

They are. As for size of breast, this has nothing to do with its ability to make milk; a mother with a small bra size can be just as successful as her more amply endowed neighbor.

Inverted or flat nipples may cause some difficulty unless some care has been given them beforehand. But with patience and ingenuity you will find you are able to manage quite well. For more detailed information on inverted nipples, see pages 29-30.

Won't Nursing Spoil the Shape of My Breasts?

On the contrary; if breastfeeding has any effect, it will be to improve your figure. The bugbear here is the fear of developing pendulous breasts. Proper support during pregnancy and the avoidance of obesity (both needed whether you plan to nurse or not) are all that is necessary to keep you in good shape.

Could I Have Inherited An Inability to Breastfeed?

No, the fact that your mother, or your grandmother for that matter, thought she was unable to nurse her babies is no reason for you to think so too. Your equipment is entirely independent of hers. Furthermore, she was probably able to nurse whether she thought so or not.

Although you are able to nurse just by virtue of being a woman, the assurance with which you approach breastfeeding could be adversely affected by outside influence, if you let it. If your mother nursed her babies and is happy that you plan to do the same, probably all will be well. However, listening to a misinformed though well-meaning relative or friend has misled many an unsure girl into thinking that she, too, just didn't have what it takes to make a go of breastfeeding. Such outside influences, which can be tremendously strong, are known as "social pressures." Do yourself and your baby a favor and turn a deaf ear to the would-be discouragers. If they can't say anything encouraging, don't listen to them.

Can a Woman Who Is Breast Feeding Have a Cancerous Lump in Her Breast?

It is possible, but very rare—most lumps in the breasts of nursing mothers are not cancerous.

Maybe My Milk Won't Be Rich Enough

This is virtually impossible, even in poor countries. All research on breast milk attests to the fact that if it's breast milk, it's the best milk. It has, in fact, been a common observation that babies get along quite well on the milk of mothers who themselves are starving and emaciated as a result of unfortunate circumstances.

The reason this worry sometimes arises is probably that the appearance of breast milk is deceiving. Colostrum, which

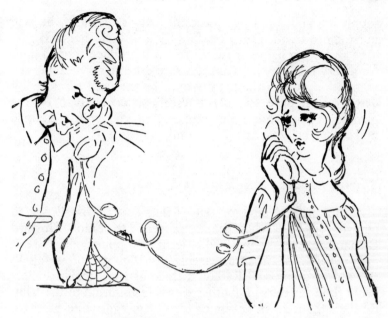

Learn to turn a deaf ear

is the fluid contained in the milk glands before the true milk comes in, is thick and yellowish; the first milk, containing some colostrum, is also rich and creamy-looking. Very soon, however, it changes to a skim-milk look, thin and almost bluish. This is the way it should look. It is perfectly adapted to your baby's digestive system and nutritional needs.

Maybe My Milk Will Be Too Rich

This is an unusual worry, but it does crop up once in a while. This is not possible either, except perhaps in the case of the very premature baby. The last sentence in the preceding section applies here as well.

What if I Don't Have Enough Milk?

You will, if you nurse your baby often enough. Ordinarily, you simply leave it up to his appetite. The more often and the longer he nurses, the more milk there will be. If the supply of milk does not meet the baby's demands, he will nurse more frequently for a few days to build it up. If you have a very big baby, or twins, you will produce enough milk for a very big baby or twins. (A rare exception to leaving the whole thing up to the baby would be the very placid baby described on page 69; in this case you do have to do the planning for a while.) But rest assured you will be able to nurse your baby, whatever his temperament.

What if My Baby Is Allergic to My Milk?

Our medical advisors tell us that no case of allergy to human milk itself has been reported. Dr. Frank Howard Richardson, well-known pediatrician, also points out: "Breast milk never causes infantile eczema, although it is often falsely accused of doing so." Rarely, a trace of a particularly allergenic food the nursing mother eats is transmitted to the baby through the milk in an intact form; e.g. egg-white proteins, which may cause sensitivity to the milk. But this is rare and is simply solved by removing the offending food from the mother's diet. If a baby who is getting nothing but breast milk (no juices, vitamins, or other supplements) develops eczema or allergic-like symptoms, look first for some substance with which he comes in contact. A few common possibilities are colored sheets, detergents, soaps and soap powders, wool, or feathers. If you yourself are taking any drugs or medicines, this might be causing the trouble. If the trouble persists, consult your physician. Allergy of any kind is never a reason for weaning the baby, and breastfeeding is the best protection against developing additional allergies from the usual food substitutes.

One baby we know of developed a bad rash, and the doctor suggested that it was eczema due to an allergy to breast milk. He advised weaning the baby. Before agreeing to take the baby off the breast, however, the mother asked for a second medical opinion. The second doctor called it diaper rash, and with a change in laundering methods and the help of a simple ointment, the rash cleared up within a week, with the baby still happily nursing. Several experiences of this sort reported by mothers, plus the opinions of our own medical advisors, have convinced us this isn't something you need to be concerned about.

Will the Milk of an Rh-Negative Mother Be Bad for Her Baby?

No, the Rh-negative mother need not hesitate to breast-feed her baby. Doctors have seen many such mothers nurse their babies with no apparent adverse reactions; even in cases where the baby has had to have transfusions, he has thrived on his mother's milk.

Will a Caesarean Affect Breastfeeding?

An operative delivery does not keep the milk from coming in. However, it should be understood that such a mother has undergone a major operation, has had an anesthetic of some sort, and is not feeling as shipshape as the mother who has had a normal labor and delivery. Her recovery will be slower, her stay in the hospital longer.

If your baby has to be delivered by Caesarean section, you may need to have more patience and persistence than the mother who has had a normal delivery. However, if you follow the usual suggestions for helping the milk supply, there is no reason why you cannot nurse successfully. In fact, we have talked and corresponded with many mothers who have done so. One of them has had three babies by Caesarean section and successfully nursed all three. Women who have done this report that nursing the baby is a most restful occupation for a convalescing mother. It also contributes to the healing of the uterine scar.

How About Twins?

You'll manage! You may have read a few years ago about a study of mothers of twins made by Dr. Benjamin Spock. If so, you will remember he found, to his surprise and pleasure, that the mothers who nursed both babies completely were the best organized, time-wise, and at an earlier date than the mothers who partially nursed, or even bottle-fed their babies. The mothers at the top of the list nursed the twins simultaneously. Interesting, isn't it?

Our own Viola Lennon recently had twins (her sixth and seventh babies). Also, many of the mothers with whom we have kept in touch have had twins and breastfed them successfully. We will tell you how they managed in Chapter 6 (pages 85-88).

Some Babies Are Premature—What Then?

The mother who delivers her baby prematurely has a special situation which requires special handling. But don't think for a minute you won't be able to nurse your little premie. We know a number of mothers who have. In fact, the premie benefits even more than the full-term baby from the warm closeness associated with breastfeeding. The degree of prematurity and other considerations will affect the handling of the premie during the early weeks of his life. In Chapter 7 we outline the various possibilities and suggest how you and your doctor may work out the best plan for your own little fellow (see pages 91-93).

What if I Get Sick?

You won't need to worry about having to stop nursing if you come down with such ailments as a cold or the flu, the most common ills you are likely to pick up while the baby is small. The baby, having been close to you till now, has undoubtedly been exposed to these germs before you even knew they were around. As you already know, breast milk is good protection for your baby against infections. From your point of view, it is certainly a lot more restful than bottle feeding with all the work that involves, and the more rest you get, the speedier your recovery.

As for more serious illnesses or emergencies, perhaps even involving hospitalization, your doctor will help you work out the best plan in the particular circumstances. Some mothers have been permitted to take their babies into the hospital with them. In only the most unusual circumstances would it be necessary for you to stop breastfeeding permanently; meanwhile, something can be worked out to carry you and the baby over this trying situation (see pages 97-98).

What if the Baby Gets Sick?

Your breastfed baby is not as likely to get sick as is his bottle-fed neighbor. If he should, however, continued breastfeeding is by far the best thing for him in practically all instances (see pages 104-107).

Do Menstrual Periods Affect Nursing?

First let's get clearly in mind the relation between breastfeeding, the resumption of menstrual periods, and ovulation. While a mother is *wholly* breastfeeding (no solids or supplements), she will most likely not menstruate at all. In fact, the average nursing mother will not have a period for about seven to fifteen months after giving birth (see pages 9-10). When she does begin to have menstrual periods, at least one and often several of these will be without ovulation, or sterile, in most cases. Only a fraction of 1 per cent of women are likely to conceive while wholly breastfeeding before having any periods.

Some women, however, do not experience postponement of their periods, and they will naturally wonder about the effect of menstruation on nursing.

Menstruation is no reason to give up breastfeeding, since it does not affect the quality of the milk in any way. If you tend to be quite nervous just before or during your period, you might possibly experience some difficulty for a day or so during that time—tension does sometimes affect the let-down reflex so that the milk will not begin to flow as easily as it ordinarily does. However, the milk hasn't disappeared, and the interference with the let-down is only temporary. Just continue to nurse your baby often, while you make every effort to relax, for your own sake as well as the baby's.

Could I Be Too Nervous to Nurse?

Nervousness of the mother, when carried to extremes, can hold back her milk in the way we have just described, but *it does not diminish the supply*. If you're the type who tends to be high-strung, your let-down may sometimes be slower in starting. It will help to recognize that you need have no real worries as regards the milk supply. Recognize also that with motherhood you need to adopt a generally more relaxed attitude toward life. It makes sense, too, to try to avoid situations that you know might upset you; your husband can be helpful here (see Chapter 8). For specific suggestions on ways of lessening tension while you are nursing, see pages 77-78.

What if I Don't Have the Let-Down Reflex?

Let's first explain just what the let-down reflex is. The let-down reflex is a natural, involuntary action. What happens is that the sucking of the baby normally causes a hormone called oxytocin to enter the blood stream. This acts on the tiny milk sacs in your breast so that they push or squeeze the milk out into the bigger ducts in the breast where the baby can suck it out. Incidentally, this oxytocin is a pretty powerful hormone; it also acts to make the uterus contract, which is one reason why breastfeeding soon after delivery is so good for you.

Sometimes just hearing your baby cry, seeing him, or thinking about him, will start the milk letting-down. You don't have to do anything consciously to start it. Possibly you will notice a tingling sensation in the breast at the beginning of nursing, or sometimes between feedings. That's it.

It is true that tension and worry could interfere with your let-down, from time to time; but there is no such thing as not having it. When you are relaxed and confident, it will happen, as surely as day follows night.

Isn't It too Hard to Nurse If There Are Older Children?

Heavens, no. It is when you do have other children to care for that you most appreciate how much easier it is to have a baby at the breast than to cope with making formula, sterilizing bottles, and so on. It takes two hands to give a baby a bottle properly; breastfeeding takes only one. A nursing mother has a free hand which can wipe a nose, dry a tear, hold a book, help a child dress, or just give him a hug and a love. Once in a while, nursing is a fine time for a story for the other little ones. Then they can look forward to it as their time, too.

Older children, even the toddler, can be a great help to you. You let them do the little errands around the house that can save you steps—and let them feel their importance in the family as they help. There is added joy in "sharing" your tiny one with his brothers and sisters.

If it's a question of "What can I tell the other children?" or "How can I explain? What will they think?"—this is a concern you should set aside at once. Breastfeeding your baby is the right and proper thing to do, and what better time for your children to learn this than right now? Our children accept breastfeeding for what it is: a nice, easy, cozy, comforting way to feed a baby. They learn that this is what breasts are for. Our sons realize this is one important difference between men and women: mommies have breasts so they can feed their babies; daddies don't feed the baby, so they don't need breasts. Our little daughters look forward to the day when they, too, can nurse their babies. In this manner, motherly acts and feelings rub off on these little mothers of the future. How many of us have seen our three- or four-year-old crooning softly to her dolly, clasped close to its "mommy's" flat little chest. Here is where the first young stirrings of mothering appear; where today's children learn to become tomorrow's parents.

What if I Get Pregnant Again?

This is possible, of course, although breastfeeding practically always postpones pregnancy for some time (see pages 9-10). It is most unusual for the mother to become pregnant while she is *completely* nursing her baby, without solids or supplements. If you do become pregnant again while you are nursing, this doesn't mean you must wean the baby immediately. He will usually be taking plenty of solids by this time and will taper off gradually by himself. Of course, you have to make particularly certain that you are getting enough rest to prevent fatigue and that you are eating well. This is for your own sake; Nature sees to it that both babies are getting what they need.

There is more on weaning in Chapter 9. The point to be made here is that you *can* continue to nurse your older baby when you become pregnant again, so let him stay a baby as long as he likes, and enjoy him. You have plently of time to wean him gradually and easily.

What If My Baby Teethes Early?

The commonest worry with early teethers is biting. Sore gums do sometimes cause a teething baby to bite toward the end of a feeding. However, "ouch!" from the mother, as she quickly removes him from the breast, if only momentarily, usually puts an end to biting. Seeing that he has something else to teethe on is also helpful.

In older babies, if playful nipping seems to occur often at the same feeding each day, the little one probably no longer needs that feeding. Try eliminating it and see what happens.

Then, Can Nothing Keep Me from Nursing My Baby?

We can't go quite that far. If, when the baby is born, you should have either whooping cough or active open tuberculosis, you would definitely not be allowed to nurse your baby. You and the baby would have to be separated until you were well. After that, you would try to give your baby the very best mothering you could manage without breastfeeding, remembering that every baby needs the warm closeness of being held by his mother, especially while feeding.

Some babies with cleft palate cannot suck, but they can still be given mother's milk. Lee M. used an electric pump for eight months to express the milk for her eighth child, giving it to her in a special bottle. Subsequently, the baby was in the best of health before undergoing the necessary surgery. Recovery was quick, and along with her brothers and sisters, Theresa is enjoying the happy childhood which follows easily and naturally a babyhood blessed with good mothering.

Chapter 5

Your Baby Arrives

At the hospital you may need to be prepared to assert yourself, in a nice way. Luckily, more and more hospitals are realizing the importance of breastfeeding, and the nurses are giving more help and encouragement to the nursing mother. On the other hand, not all hospitals are ideally set up to be of the greatest possible help. In such hospitals you can expect a few raised eyebrows from some hospital personnel when they find out that you've "taken the notion" to nurse your baby. Just cheerfully and firmly let them know you really mean it. Take the attitude that you are being quite progressive. (A recent Harvard study indicates a trend back to breastfeeding headed up by the better-educated women.) If your hospital happens to be one of the more old-fashioned ones, offering little help to the nursing mother, don't let them get you down, and plan to go home as soon as you're able.

If you happen to land in one of those wonderful modern hospitals with rooming-in, or one which goes all out to help a nursing mother and her baby, three cheers! (Rooming-in means keeping the baby in the same room with his mother instead of in a central nursery with the other babies.)

No Supplement; Frequent Nursing

Your doctor can be a big help if he's enthusiastic about breastfeeding. He can leave orders in the nursery that your baby is not to be given any bottles between nursings, even in the first few days prior to the coming in of the breast milk. He may do this even if he's lukewarm about breastfeeding, if you ask him to do it. So do ask him ahead of time and remind him about it, if he agrees. It won't hurt to mention casually to the nurse that you're glad your baby isn't getting any formula—since you'll be completely breastfeeding him, any formula given now *could* lead to his developing an allergy to cow's milk when that is reintroduced into his diet several months later. The nursing staff may not know this fact about allergies, and through busy forgetfulness, or simply out of the goodness of their hearts, they may think they are doing your baby a kindness by giving him a bottle or two during those first days before your milk comes in. Knowing this allergy fact may help them remember the doctor's orders.

Your doctor may also be able to arrange to have your baby brought to you at least every three hours while you are in the hospital, and certainly for at least one night feeding.

These two measures are very helpful if they can be arranged, because the supplementary formula is one of the greatest deterrents to establishing a good milk supply, and frequent nursing is one of the greatest helps. You see, the milk supply is regulated by what the baby takes. The more he nurses, the more milk there will be. If he's given a bottle as well, he'll gradually take less and less from the breast and the supply will diminish.

Another reason for encouraging frequent nursing during these first days following your baby's birth is that this is the period during which your breasts are supplying him with his first nourishment, colostrum. Colostrum is the yellowish fluid which your body has been making during the latter months of your pregnancy. It's what you have been hand-expressing if you have followed our suggestions for prenatal nipple care (see page 28), or you may have noticed a few drops of it on your nipples occasionally during the last few months before the baby was born. The colostrum is in increased supply right after delivery, and it remains an ingredient in your milk for about ten days. Colostrum is especially designed for the newborn baby. It is easier for him to digest because of its lower fat and carbohydrate content. Also, it is even richer in immunity factors than the milk. Finally, it has a slightly laxative effect, clearing out the meconium (the dark green or blackish matter discharged from the newborn baby's bowels) and in general readying his digestive tract for the milk he'll be getting in a few days.

Do not be misled or discouraged by the baby's not gaining weight during the first ten days or so. It is normal for the newborn of all species to lose weight following birth. In the human it takes about one to three weeks for the baby to regain his birth weight, whether breastfed or bottle-fed.

Don't Take Any Formula Home with You

If it's not in the house, you won't be tempted to use it in a moment of doubt. On the other hand, one mother told us the formula she was given to take home made dandy pancakes for the family. If you are both strong-minded and thrifty, you may want to follow her example.

If you are already home and the baby has been given some supplement, you can stop now, and your milk supply will build up again, perhaps with the temporary aid of more frequent nursings.

Shots and Pills and Such

If you should be given shots or pills to "dry you up," don't worry about it, though you might try to avoid them. These are usually a routine carried over from the mother who doesn't breastfeed. This medication, usually a form of stilbestrol, is given to reduce the discomfort of engorged breasts; if you continue to nurse your baby, it will not hinder your milk flow. In fact, we know of several doctors who routinely give stilbestrol to their nursing mothers believing that, by reducing the engorgement, this medication will make the mother more comfortable and thus cause her milk to come in more easily. At any rate, with or without it, you can nurse your baby.

There is a new drug which is specifically intended to assist breastfeeding. It is syntocinon, which is used in the form of a nasal spray. Its purpose is to act as the natural hormone oxytocin ordinarily does, which is to bring on the let-down reflex and help get the milk flow started. This might prove helpful in some few cases, if the mother is very doubtful of her ability to breastfeed, or if she is so tense and nervous that her let-down is a bit slow. It should, of course, be used only on a doctor's prescription.

Actually, some doctors feel that since both of these, stilbestrol and syntocinon, are hormonal drugs, they could have unwelcome side-effects. Anyhow, they only do for you what Nature is already doing. It's usually better to trust in your natural womanly make-up to do the job for you. Remember, mothers have been nursing babies for thousands of years before these artificial "aids" were discovered.

How Long to Nurse

You may be cautioned by more than one person while in the hospital not to let the baby nurse too long or too often for fear of getting sore nipples. Don't cut the nursing too short on this account, particularly if you have followed the suggestions for nipple care during pregnancy; but it might be wise to limit nursing to five or ten minutes on each side at each feeding for the first few days. Keep in mind that more frequent, shorter nursing periods are easier on the nipples. The important thing the first week after delivery is to stimulate the milk supply. Many women never get sore nipples no matter how much their babies nurse. Some do, however, and we have mentioned what to do to help avoid this (page 28). We will also give you some suggestions later about coping with this condition if it should occur (see page 98). What we want to emphasize here is that it won't do any good to keep the nipples from getting sore and then not have enough milk for the baby, so let's take first things first.

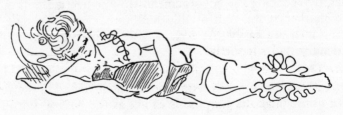

Nipple Cleansing

The hospital will have some routine for cleaning the nipples and keeping the baby's wrappings from contact with your sheets. The reason for this is the necessity for great care in the hospital, where many different people are assembled. We have found soap, alcohol, and tincture of benzoin to be very drying to the nipples. However, if your doctor feels that this "sterile" technique is necessary, by all means follow it while in the hospital. At home, with just the "family" germs around, it won't be necessary. Your baby is immune to what you are immune to. This is part of the inheritance he gets from you through the placental transmission of antibodies. He does not have the same immunity to strangers' germs.

Sleeping or Screaming

Very often, because hospital schedules don't coincide too well with baby's appetite, he will be either sound asleep or screaming his head off when feeding time comes around. We don't know which is more disconcerting! If he is sleeping, try gently to awaken him; rough handling is very disturbing to the newborn. Joggle him gently and place his cheek against your breast. If he doesn't wake up, let it go; it won't hurt him to sleep through a feeding, especially if he is being brought to you every three hours. If you know the hospital routine calls for bringing the baby in at longer intervals, and perhaps not at all during the night, you might try a little harder to rouse him—but never at all roughly. *Please* don't snap the soles of his feet with your fingernail.

If he is crying very hard, it may call for a bit of patience to quiet him. Talk to him, hold him gently and securely close to you, and he'll soon stop. Easy does it.

Your nurse may know all about breastfeeding and be friendly and supportive; if so, she will be giving you little practical hints about handling the small bundle she brings you every three hours or so. In case she has no suggestions for you, the above points are the important ones to remember in the hospital. For the rest, follow the same how-to suggestions you will be using at home (see Chapter 6).

Your Hospital and You

Like doctors, hospitals vary in their practices, and we can't tell you exactly what you will find in yours. We have suggested that you talk this over with your doctor, so that he can give you some idea of what to expect. If you do run into considerable opposition, don't antagonize the hospital personnel by throwing your weight around and telling them how to run their hospital. You can't win. Be firm about breastfeeding, but otherwise go slow on trying to buck established routines; smile and smile, and get out of there as fast as your doctor will let you. Do write a nice letter to the hospital directors stating your views, after you get home. Such letters often carry a lot of weight. You may make it easier for the next breastfeeding mother delivering in that hospital, and—who knows?—you may find a delightfully changed atmosphere on *your* next visit.

There is one other thing you can do. It may be the custom in your hospital to leave a little gift with the nurses, such as a box of candy. Whether or not such a gift is customary, you can certainly also leave with them a copy of the La Leche League pamphlet for nurses (see page 155). It's a nice way to say "thank you" to them and to let them know that this kind of information is available. Many hospitals would be glad to have this and might be encouraged to get a quantity of them from the League for all their nurses.

And away you go from the hospital. Whatever the ups and downs of your hospital stay, *when you get your baby home you will be able to nurse him*. Thousands of mothers have done so in similar circumstances. Providentially, the hospital picture is changing rapidly as more and more hospitals adopt more up-to-date practices in their maternity wards. The probability is that yours will be neither the best nor the worst in this respect. Whatever it is, appreciate it for the service it offers and know that, whatever your hospital experience has been, you *can* nurse your baby.

Chapter 6

"How-To"

In this chapter we are going to mention some specific ways of taking care of your baby, and yourself, which we and hundreds of mothers we have talked to and advised have found comfortable and easy Use them as friendly tips from one mother to another—things to try, in a relaxed, easygoing way, as you learn the special ways of handling your own little individualist.

Babies Are to Love

Through it all, remember that babies are to love. Spend less time on complicated bathing, dressing, and feeding routines, and more on what doctors call TLC—"tender, loving care"—which the very best medical authorities recognize as being the prime need of babies.

"Diapering" is another way of showing your love and attention to your baby. Your goal here is his comfort. He should be snug and warm when put to bed. The simpler the clothing, the better for him. Fairly frequent changes of wet diapers, when he is awake, plus restricting the use of rubber or plastic pants to dress-up occasions, should prevent diaper rash. Forget the darling bonnet or the fancy jacket for everyday living. This is a baby to be loved, not a doll to dress up.

During the early months, baby will be spending most of his waking time with you. (Incidentally, some babies sleep very little during the day.) The tiny baby needs to be with his mother, to feel her warmth and closeness, even the rhythms of her breathing and heartbeat to which he has been accustomed before birth. As the weeks go by and he becomes more aware of the world around him, he needs to be included often in the family group. Many people have noticed the difference in the very early alertness and response of the baby whose basket or cradle is moved from room to room with

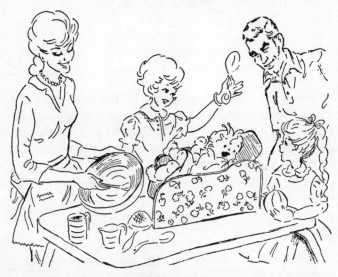

He'll want to be near you much of the time

the family, and who is talked to and sung to and smiled at as compared with the baby who spends most of the early months of his life alone in the bedroom, behind the bars of his crib.

So, whatever else you do, you will want to have baby with you most of the time as a matter of course. Naturally, you won't be holding him in your arms every minute, though you will be doing that, too, both when you are nursing him and between times as he needs it. Above all, you will just want to be there because what your baby needs most of all is you. No one else can take your place; no one else will make him as happy. To him, there is nobody quite like mother.

Just a reminder here about those little extras we suggested, which would make it easier to have baby near you.

The rocker, the cradle on wheels, and so on can be most welcome in any household.

Now, we will get on with our specific suggestions, beginning at the moment when you are first handed your small miraculous bundle. If this is your first baby, you will probably be a little scared of him; don't worry. As you try different ways of holding him and caring for him, always be very slow and gentle. You will soon be an old hand at it. Maybe you will discover little "tricks of the trade" we haven't mentioned; and later on, when you have time, perhaps you will write us about them.

How to Hold the Baby to Nurse Him

Whichever position you find most comfortable for you and the baby is the best for you. During the early weeks, you may find it more relaxing and convenient to lie down while you nurse the baby. Certainly this is the thing to do for those middle-of-the-night suppers, so that you can doze back to sleep while he is nursing. Later on, you may prefer to sit in a chair or in a corner of the sofa for most of his feedings during the day.

In the beginning, when you are lying down, and you are going to nurse your baby on the right side, lie down on that side, put your right arm up over the baby's head or under it, whichever is more comfortable for you. With the left arm, bring the baby toward you *till his cheek is touching your breast,* with the nipple next to his mouth. He will turn his head toward it, for this is the way he is built, and open his mouth. When he does, pull him in a bit closer, just enough so he can get the nipple into his mouth and suck. For nursing on the left side, reverse all this. If you pull his legs close to you, it angles his body enough to keep his nose free. This keeps him warm and cozy besides.

When removing the baby from the breast, be sure to first gently press the breast away from the corner of his mouth with your finger until the suction is broken. Just pulling him off the breast can be hard on the nipple.

Sometimes a very full breast will make it difficult for the baby to grasp the nipple. This often happens at the first feeding in the morning. After several hours' sleep the breast may be quite full and hard. If the baby acts frustrated and cries and turns his head away from the breast, even though you are pretty sure he is hungry, this may very well be the reason. In such a case, you can hand-express a little milk first so as to get the flow started, as well as to get the nipple out, ready for the baby to grasp it easily. (If you have not already learned the knack of hand-expression, before the baby was born, you can easily pick it up now. See page 28.) You may also need to hold the full breast a little away from his nose if it seems to be interfering with his breathing. Just press it away slightly with your finger, enough to make an airway for him.

Here is the story of how one mother learned this the hard way:

> Rita J. went through a miserable week of a crying, frustrated baby before she realized what the trouble was. Her baby nursed happily at all other feedings, but screamed angrily at the early morning feeding. Each time she ended up resorting to formula, after which she had to hand-express her milk to get relief from her over-full breasts. Finally, she called a La Leche mother, who cleared up the mystery. She suggested that perhaps the heaviness of the full morning breast was making it impossible for the baby to grasp the nipple. Rita did as we suggested above; and from then on, she had a baby who was happy all day long, right from early morning.

Another difficulty that might come up, especially at that early morning feeding and during the first few weeks while the baby is tiny and inexperienced, is that the first milk may come spurting out, as if jet-propelled. An older baby could take this in stride, but the tiny fellow may find it just too much too soon. He may choke and gulp, and the milk may run out of his mouth instead of down his throat. If your little one is acting this way, and you know your milk is coming out quite fast, try letting the first milk run into a cup or a hanky, and let the baby take over when the flow is slowed down.

As to nursing sitting up, you will experiment until you find the most comfortable position. The only suggestion we would make is that when you are starting out you will do well to keep in mind that you are going to be in this position for a while, so arrange matters so that you can be relaxed, with none of your muscles involved in holding either yourself or the baby without support. Pillows are useful at your back, or your elbow, under the baby, or wherever you like. If you can prop your feet up, so much the better; a new mother's legs get pretty tired at first, so kick off your shoes and get your feet up if you are comfortable that way.

How Often and How Long?

In the beginning the baby will probably want to be fed about every two to three hours, with perhaps one longer stretch a day. We always hope this long stretch will happen some time between midnight and 6 A.M. The four-hour idea became firmly implanted in people's minds as a result of hospital schedules and formula feeding. Hospital schedules ended up that way because they were adapted to the convenience of the hospital and the nursing staff, rather than to the baby. Formula, because it is not as well adapted to the baby's digestive system as breast milk, takes longer to digest. Formula can also encourage overfeeding, so as to get the baby to "last" four hours. If you keep in mind that formulas and rigid schedules have nothing to do with *your* baby, it becomes quite simple. Most babies know when they need to be fed, so you'll let him decide, whether the interval is two hours, three hours, or longer.

With all babies, it is probably best to use both breasts at each feeding, certainly until the milk supply is well established. Even then, you and he may want to continue this way.

Do it like this: Give the baby one side for about ten minutes. Then, after time out for a rest, or a burp, or a change of diapers, switch over to the other side for as long as you and he like, probably twenty minutes or so, perhaps more. Next time, reverse the order, using the last-used side first and the first last. Doing the necessary diapering and burping between courses in this way means that he won't be delayed first of all in getting fed; and it also means that, after he has finished the second half of his meal, if he has fallen asleep he can be set down quietly, all warm and full. Later you may want to nurse on only one side at a feeding. Suit yourself and the baby about this.

When the Milk Comes in: "Losing" Your Milk

This isn't exactly a "how-to," but it belongs here because it will be going on when you are starting to nurse the baby and may cause you some amazement and even concern.

The milk first comes in any time from the second to the fifth or sixth day. Before that, your baby will be getting colostrum, which is also nourishing and important for him (see page 54). Many factors combine to bring your milk in sooner; the most important one is being at ease. Natural childbirth and rooming-in are usually a contribution in this direction. Getting home soon to your own familiar relaxing surroundings with the independence it gives you in being able to cuddle and nurse your baby whenever he needs it, and to be yourself, is also most helpful.

When the milk comes in, especially if it is your first baby, your breast may suddenly seem to be fairly bursting with it. Naturally, you are overjoyed and confident. But, about a week later, suddenly the milk seems to be gone. No more full feeling, no more excess milk dripping out. At this point many mothers become discouraged and really believe that they have "lost" their milk. In fact, some are convinced it never came in at all.

You see, the first coming-in of the milk is frequently, though not always, accompanied by a good deal of engorgement; that is, the breasts often swell considerably. This isn't all milk. It is rather like the marshalling of the grand army— all the forces come to the fore to get things in good working order for the months to come. There is swelling of the tissues, extra blood rushes into these veins, and all these things combine to make it seem as if you have gallons of milk. This bursting feeling and dripping milk happens most often in first-time mothers; but, as we said, some of these never experience it. Others notice it to a lesser degree. Mothers who have already had one or more babies may notice it even less. It is merely a matter of individual difference and has no real influence on the amount of milk you will have for your baby.

In the normal course of events, the engorgement subsides, and things settle down. In fact, if you have been given drying-up pills, you will likely not notice any engorgement; but with continued, regular nursing, your milk will come in as well as ever. (See page 55.) Whatever your experience may be, the capacity of your breasts to supply all the milk your baby needs is still there for the asking, and the baby has no trouble asking for it. The making of the milk is almost a continuous process; as the baby takes it out, more comes in.

So, don't be afraid you have "lost" your milk. You haven't. Just keep nursing as usual.

There may be seeming changes in the supply more than once in the weeks ahead because the supply is adjusting to your baby's needs. The more often your baby empties your breasts, the more milk you will have. If you have twins, you will have enough for twins. When the baby nurses less often and less completely (or vigorously), the amount of milk you make drops accordingly; if it drops too far to suit him, he will nurse more often and your breast will respond by making more milk. Periodically, during a growth spurt, your baby may go on a nursing binge to build up your milk supply to meet his new demands. A recent study reported in the medical journals verifies this ancient example of Nature's ability to adapt. Doctors found that if a mother's milk supply seemed to lag behind her baby's needs, increased breastfeeding over a period of forty-eight hours brought the supply up to meet the demand, and the baby was once again satisfied.

You see how it works? Unhampered by rigid schedules or supplementary foods, this is one of the best examples left in this complicated world of ours of the operation of the law of supply and demand. It takes a little while to establish a working equilibrium between baby's appetite and your milk supply, so do not get impatient. The first six weeks are sometimes the most challenging; just take it easy and let nature take its course.

Sometimes mothers are told to empty their breasts completely after each feeding by pumping out whatever milk the baby may leave. We have yet to find a mother who has a normal, healthy baby who found this necessary to a good milk supply. Most women who start this sort of pumping soon give it up because it is a great bother and quite time-consuming. If you pump, you will make more milk than your baby needs at this point, thus throwing a small monkey wrench into a delicately-balanced system that works beautifully without it. The only reason we know of for pumping is to be able to send your milk in to your own baby who has to be separated from you for some reason, or to share it with another baby in need of breast milk and unable to get it from his own mother. If you should have a baby who does not as yet suck well, as in the case of some premies, or an occasional full-term baby, you might have to pump after each feeding in order to provide sufficient stimulation to keep up your supply.

Burping the Baby

Because of the mechanics of bottle feeding, bottle-fed babies do usually swallow air that needs to be expelled if the baby is to be comfortable. This is not as true of the breastfed baby. Some breastfed babies never seem to need burping, others only in the early months. They are more likely to swallow air if they are overeager nursers, "gulpers." or at the very full breast, when the milk comes out fast. The baby who has been crying long and hard—a situation you should, of course, avoid—will naturally not nurse as calmly and placidly as the baby who is put to the breast when he first makes his needs known.

In any event, your baby may need burping. Certainly it is one of the things you try if he is fussy; but you don't need to worry about making it an inflexible part of the business of nursing. Your experiences with your own baby will be your best guide as to whether and when your baby needs burping.

Try a little gentle patting on the back when you switch from one breast to the other, or when he is through nursing. If the "bubble" doesn't come up in a few moments forget it, unless he is quite fussy and seems to like what you're doing. If he does burp, especially if he burps loudly and heartily, see if he wants a little more milk. The big bubble may have deceived him into thinking he was full when he really wasn't. If he falls asleep at the breast when being nursed peacefully, don't bother him with the burping routine. Always lay him down on his side or tummy; sometimes the right side works better than the left side. In this position the air bubble, if there is one, will probably come up spontaneously, and any milk he may spit up will run out of his mouth instead of down his throat.

Cleanliness and the Nipples

Ordinary washing care is all that is necessary for your breasts and nipples. Once you get home from the hospital, there is no need for special cleaning techniques, either before or after nursing. When you do bathe, we recommend avoiding the use of soap on the nipples; it isn't necessary. Soap is drying to the skin, and dryness encourages cracked nipples. If you are using gauze pads, or your husband's clean folded hankies to catch leaking milk, these can be changed as needed; and with a fresh bra daily your breast will be as clean as can be.

Mothers sometimes think that they have to keep on at home with the rather elaborate nipple-cleansing routines followed at the hospital. We have already mentioned that this is necessary in the hospital because, with the risks of cross-infections there from germs new to you—strangers, so to speak—everything has to be done in as sterile a manner as possible. At home, however, where for the most part you are at home with your germs and your germs are at home with you, sterility is not necessary, and you will only make yourself miserable trying to achieve it. Women who bottle feed have to take great pains to keep the formula sterile because there is a lapse of time between its preparation and the baby's feeding, so that any germs would have a chance to multiply in it unless great care is taken. *Your* milk goes directly from you to your baby.

Of course, even at home there is a possibility of your picking up a few "strange" germs on your hands—taking in a package at the door, wiping your kindergartner's runny nose, or whatever—but ordinary hand-washing will take care of that nicely. You'll probably instinctively use a little extra care in this respect the first month or so, and that will be fine.

Is Baby Getting Enough?

If you are following his needs instead of a rigid schedule, and he is happy about it, he is getting enough. One way to reassure yourself that the baby is getting enough to eat is to note whether he is thriving and putting on weight. One way to reassure yourself that the baby is getting enough fluid is to check the number of wet diapers. If he has six or eight or more wet diapers a day, he is doing fine. Occasionally, water may be advantageous on excessively hot days.

Weighing the Baby

You or the doctor will probably weigh the baby from time to time, because it is one of the most concrete ways of measuring his physical progress. Once a month is usually often enough. An average of a pound a month, or four to seven ounces a week, is a good gain. Anything over that is extra. If your baby is gaining less than a pound a month, though, don't jump to the conclusion that your milk isn't good enough. (See pages 44-45.) By all means, continue to nurse him, stepping up the number of feedings, from three hours to two, or even from two to more often, for a day or so. Remember the rule—the more he empties the breast, the more milk there will be.

Don't try to find out how many ounces of milk the baby is getting from you by weighing him before and after each feeding. Babies don't usually take the same amount of milk at each feeding, so mother may worry needlessly. The baby knows if he is getting enough. If he isn't he will nurse more often, and this will bring the supply up. If he is, what does it matter exactly how many ounces he takes at any one feeding? The whole routine of weighing "before and after" is cumbersome; it means making the baby wait beforehand, when he is hungry and impatient to be fed, and jiggling him around afterward when he wants to be quiet. It makes a big production out of each feeding, and neither you nor the baby have anything to gain from that.

Weighing the Extra-Placid Baby, or the "Sleeper"

Every so often you will find a very placid, polite baby who regularly sleeps for four or five hours at a time, is not too urgent about demanding food when he does awaken, and nurses rather leisurely. As time goes on, he may seem to get even quieter, and you think, "Such a good baby. He's certainly doing well." Then comes the surprise when you take him to the doctor for his check-up and find he isn't gaining. We don't know what makes some babies behave this way, but we do know that you have to encourage them to nurse often, and perhaps even coax them a bit to stay awake and nurse longer; always gently, of course. With this kind of baby, you have to do the deciding for a while. It might be a good idea to follow his weight more closely, about once a week, not to make sure he is gaining at a standard rate, or weighing a certain number of pounds at a certain age, but to assure yourself that he is gaining, even though slowly and perhaps rather unevenly. If his weight seems to be staying stationary, or even dropping a bit, for longer than a week or so, you would want to increase your tactful efforts to encourage him to nurse more often, at least every two hours with possibly one longer stretch a day. In some very exceptional cases, the doctor may want to supplement the baby's diet.

Fat Babies vs. Thin Ones

We want to stress again that you don't ordinarily need to bother with checking weight in this way except in the case of the unusually sleepy, quiet infant who is regularly going four hours or more between feedings, who is nursing indifferently, and who does not seem to be thriving. Healthy, happy babies come in all shapes and sizes; individual differences are to be accepted as a matter of course. Very fat babies are no healthier than thin ones; in many cases they are less so, since overweight can be a problem for the infant as well as for the adult, and doctors are becoming increasingly concerned about the extra-rich diets some bottle-fed and some solid-fed babies are getting. On the other hand, if you have a completely breastfed baby who seems overly fat, you can be reassured by British physician Charlotte Naish who states it is impossible to gain too much on breast milk. "The tissues built up from a diet so perfectly adapted to the babies' needs cannot in any

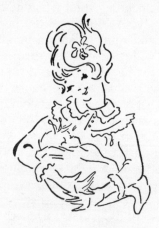

way be abnormal." If your young baby is nursing every two or three hours, if he has bowel movements (see next section) and lots of wet diapers, above all, if he has good skin elasticity and color, bright eyes, and an alert manner, don't worry about his weight.

Bowel Movements

The breastfed baby's stool differs a good deal from that of the formula-fed infant's. The odor, unlike that of the bottle-fed baby's, is mild and not unpleasant. Happily enough, he does not get constipated. The breast milk contains enough water for his needs. (Constipation, incidentally, does not have anything to do with whether a baby strains to pass his stool, nor with a time interval. Some breastfed babies go for five to seven days and have perfectly normal, though naturally profuse, stools. He is constipated only if he has a hard, dry stool.) The breastfed baby's stool is usually quite loose and unformed, often of a pea-soup consistency. It is yellow to yellow-green to brownish in color. Sometimes there is just a stain on the diaper. The frequency varies somewhat from baby to baby and even from week to week with the same baby. At first he may have one bowel movement with every diaper change. This is definitely not a diarrhea in the breast-fed baby. Or, perhaps, he may have only two or three larger ones a week, or sometimes only one a week. So you see, there is room for considerable variation among perfectly normal breastfed babies. Even an occasional green, watery stool is not an indication for worry in the otherwise healthy baby. (Remember that bowel movements change in color after exposure to the air.) If your baby does have a diarrhea, this rarely means you must stop nursing him. He may have a mild cold or some other illness, in which case breastfeeding is still best. If the sick baby can take any food at all, your milk is best for him.

Why Is He Crying?

Nothing disturbs a mother as much as hearing her baby cry. Strange, but true. Your baby's cry is *meant* to be disturbing. It is his most important means of communication. It means he wants you to help him, to come to his rescue, that something is bothering him, or hurting or frightening him. Babies are sometimes fretful for reasons that you cannot immediately discover. You know there is a reason for his crying. He either wants something or needs something. The tiny baby's wants and needs are one and the same. But, even if you can't seem to calm him right away, don't get upset. If you do, your baby will soon have two needs: the one that was making him cry in the first place, and the need for a calm, loving mother. So, take it slow and easy. Remember, in handling any tiny baby, you have to move slowly and gently and quietly. Fast, jerky motions and loud noises startle him. If he is already upset for some reason, you need to be extra careful in handling him gently and soothingly.

After you have changed him, fed him, and done all the usual things, ask yourself these questions: "Have I had a big day? done something extra tiring? left the baby with someone else? had any upsetting incidents?" These might give you a clue to his behavior, since he is very sensitive to your moods and feelings and absences. If fatigue or tension are what is bothering your little one, he and you are apt to find the late afternoon a particularly trying time. Try lying down to nurse him. Chances are you will both relax and he will slide off to sleep. The half-hour or hour rest will do you good, too.

Your baby may have a burp that won't come up. Try to help him with it. Or it may be that he is lonesome for you. He can't know that you are right there unless he feels you. You might as well be in Timbuctoo as on the other side of the room, as far as he is concerned.

Here is where you may run head-on into one of the older notions we talked about earlier, and it may be advanced very persuasively by Grandma or a well-meaning friend. This notion is that if the baby is well fed, warm, dry, and generally comfortable, cries when you put him down, but soothes when you hold him, you should put him down gently but firmly to cry it out, for fear of "spoiling" him.

You can't spoil a tiny baby. On the contrary, his emotional needs are just as strong, and just as important, as his physical needs; and you are doing him an equally damaging disservice if you ignore them. Your baby's need of wanting to feel his mother close, of wanting to be cuddled in her arms, needs to be met as fully and lovingly as his needs to be fed, kept warm, and dry, and so on. So, if he stops his crying when you pick him up and hold him, just keep on holding him for a while and be happy that you are there to satisfy this important need of your infant. Don't be afraid to "baby" the baby.

These are other things you might try too, in a relaxed, cheerful way. Keep his little cradle or carrier close to you so you can reach over and rock or pat or joggle him gently every now and then. Or, you may find that, after you have held him, wrapped snugly, in an unhurried way for a while, he will settle down with a pacifier. Lay him down blanket and all, since often the shock of a cold bedsheet against his head is enough to start him crying again. We repeat "wrap him snugly," because this is often a good way of keeping your tiny baby happy. Think about how he was living before he was born. You can see how imitating that warm snugness may help him feel more secure in the big impersonal world in which he is separated from you part of the time.

There are three periods when mothers most often report extra fussiness in their babies. The first usually occurs shortly after you arrive home from the hospital. This often corresponds with a reduction in the engorgement you experienced when your milk first came in. This, coupled with

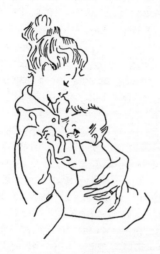

Sometimes cuddling is all that's needed

the fact that the baby has perhaps become conditioned to "crying for his supper" in the hospital, might lead you to fear that you have lost your milk, or that you just won't be able to cope with everything now that you are on your own. Read over the section on page 64 on losing your milk and also the one (page 15) on planning ahead to make life simple. Your husband would do well to read over the chapter especially for him. His calm reassurance and encouragement are important to you now. He can help keep the visitors to a minimum, and you can both accept with thanks the offers of hot meals sent in for the first few days. All these things combine to make life easier and happier for you and your baby.

The second fussy period comes when the baby is about six weeks old. What sometimes happens is that the baby is taking a growth spurt, as babies do, and temporarily his appetite gets ahead of the milk supply. Nurse the baby just as often as he seems to want it, even if it is every hour or two. When he is nursing this often, it isn't long before the milk production is stepped up to meet the increased need, the interval between nursings lengthens out again, and baby regains his sunny disposition.

When your baby is three months old, more or less, the third fussy period arrives. Here again, this is due at least in part to the same kind of jump in appetite we referred to above. Again, increased nursing will generally take care of this difficulty, since it is still a bit early for most healthy babies to have to start solids.

Another factor in the three-month fussy period, which you may or may not run into with your baby, is that he is beginning to stay awake longer and take a greater interest in the world around him. Fussing may then indicate a need for company and action, rather than hunger. Keep him in the center of activity, securely propped on the kitchen table or on a blanket on the floor where he can really stretch out. He enjoys music, movement, people going by. He tires quickly of one position, and he thrives on change and variety.

Some new babies seem to cry a lot all during the first few months of life, no matter what you do. Of course, it is especially hard to be relaxed and easygoing with such a baby, but you will both be happier if you are. Do all you can for him; wrap him snugly, walk with him, talk to him, sing to him, rock him. Dedicate yourself to him in a most loving way. Whatever you try, do it in a leisurely, unhurried way, calmly and soothingly. You can be sure that whatever solace you are able to give him will help him come through this trying period more happily and with a more solid foundation of love and security, to build on during the months and years ahead.

Generally, the observant and attentive mother will quickly learn the varied language of the cry. She will be able to differentiate the cry of hunger, of tiredness, of frustration, of pain, of discomfort just as she has learned to differentiate the unspoken words of her husband or friends.

The "Colicky" Baby

When a tiny baby has long periods of hard crying, and seems to be in some sort of physical discomfort for no apparent reason that you or your doctor can discover, he is often said to be colicky.

"Colic" is a catchall word meaning essentially "loud, persistent screaming for undetermined reasons." As many causes of colic are put forth as there are doctors who have studied it. As far back as sixty years ago, colic was referred to in one widely used pediatric text as "a scientifically inaccurate and unsatisfactory term which serves such a useful purpose in practice and covers so well a multitude of abdominal pains that it maintains its place in our medical books." The same loose definition could apply today; doctors still seem to know little or nothing about the true cause of this kind of crying. The general feeling is that it is related to some difficulty with digestion, since the baby seems to be in some sort of pain, and relief often comes with a change in feeding routine or an enema. However, since a baby in pain or discomfort from *any* cause is often consoled by frequent nursing, the pacifier, walking or rocking by the mother, this really proves nothing.

As we well know, physical pain, especially digestive disturbances, can be related to, or aggravated by, emotional distress or upsets. Just as nervous tension in the adult leads to digestive distress, a similar sort of tension could well be the cause of pain or discomfort in the tiny baby.

Perhaps the best guess is that some babies have more delicate digestive systems than others and that this factor combined with tensions and stress introduced from the outside is the likeliest cause of colic.

What to do about it? Certainly calm, gentle handling by the mother is essential. The suggestion has been made by many doctors that frequent, small feedings, geared to the baby's smaller intestinal tract, are easier for him to handle than fewer, larger feedings. Since colic usually subsides after the baby reaches the age of about three months, it has been thought that by that time he has matured enough to be able to cope somewhat better with whatever the outside world has to offer, particularly with his feedings. Meanwhile, your gentle, loving ministrations will help ease him through this period. It will help you be relaxed and calm to know that your breast milk is the best possible diet for him, and that the warm closeness of the nursing relationship is the best possible situation for easing stresses and tensions.

Overfeeding

This can sometimes happen with your breastfed baby. The kind of baby who is most apt to be overfed is the fussy, active baby whom you interpret to be hungry all the time. If you go along with this interpretation and nurse him oftener than every two hours, he only gets fussier and more restless instead of calming down. Here's the pattern: shortly after nursing he will start to howl, chew his fist, and suck on anything he can get hold of. So you try nursing him again, but he's already had as much as he can hold and he may simply spit up and howl again. Such a baby usually does not want or need more milk. He has other needs. One of them may be the need for more sucking. Often only one breast at a feeding is enough for this baby. Instead of nursing him again, try that remarkable old invention, the pacifier. Wrap him snugly and warmly and hold him while he's getting settled. If he doesn't like the pacifier at all, let him nurse again on the emptier side. No harm in that unless you have sore nipples. (If you do use a pacifier, remember that it may only pacify a symptom. It is not the best solution for all types of crying.)

How can you tell whether more sucking is what he wants, instead of more food? You can't tell for sure until you try, but if the baby who is acting as if he were starved spits up a good deal, has good bowel movements (see page 70) and plenty of wet diapers, and seems to be gaining extra fast, we would suggest one of two things: to feed him not oftener than every two or three hours, letting him suck on the pacifier between times; or to nurse him at very frequent intervals, using only one breast at a nursing. This latter method has the effect of giving him more sucking for less food, and making him suck more for his food. Try one method for a few days and then the other, giving him time to straighten out if he will. And perhaps try burping him oftener. Above all, don't get upset because, as you know, this only adds to his troubles and makes them worse. Remember, what works for one baby may not do at all for another; here, as with everything else, your own special baby has his own special behavior and may require his own special solution.

Nervous or Just Plain Tired?

This seems a good time to talk a little about the state of your nerves. If your baby happens to be one of those fussy, active ones, you may find it hard to follow our advice to relax and take it easy. If so, you have our sympathy, because we've had this kind of baby too; and we know how trying it can be. Here are a couple of suggestions to help you relax if you and the baby are giving each other the jitters.

We're taking it for granted that you have taken to heart our remarks about the baby being more important than the house, so you aren't worrying about getting all the chores done on time or keeping the house in immaculate order.

Still, maybe you've had a hard day, or something has happened to upset you, and you find yourself tense and jittery just when it's time to feed the baby and you especially want to feel calm. Take a breather and just relax for a while. Joan S. told us that she found it most relaxing just to sit down for a while with a glass of beer or a highball. If you're not averse to such things, you might try that. Another high-strung gal found that it helped to pick up a book or magazine and settle down to read with the baby at the breast. Some mothers have found that just stretching out for ten minutes or so before feeding time with a cup of coffee or something was a wonderful help.

You know, you could be hungry, too. How long since your last meal? Why not fix yourself a sandwich and glass of milk or cup of tea, and have a snack along with the baby? Of course, the old standby, which you will use most of all during the early weeks before you're completely back to par, is to take the baby with you and crawl into bed for a nap. You'll probably fall asleep while he's nursing, and so will he when he's had enough. This is especially recommended for the late afternoon, when life is apt to crowd in on both you and the baby.

Use your own best judgment, remembering that babies (and the rest of the family too) need and appreciate a relaxed mother.

Leaking?

One thing you may find rather a nuisance at times during the first weeks is that you may *leak* a little at inopportune moments. Especially if it is nearly time for a feeding, the sight or sound or even the thought of your baby may trigger the let-down reflex, and somewhat to your dismay you will realize that a few drops of milk, sometimes more, are leaking from your breasts. Or, when you're nursing from one side, you may start dripping from the other.

This never happens to some mothers. If you do experience it, it may be so slight as to cause you no inconvenience. Depending on the frequency and the amount of the leaking, you will take whatever common-sense measures are needed. Especially during the early weeks, it is very common to leak from one side while nursing on the other. Most of us find we prefer to let this happen the first few weeks—it relieves the feeling of fullness so nicely. Use a hanky or diaper to absorb the milk. After that, especially if you are out somewhere with the baby and want to rejoin the company reasonably dry, you will probably prefer to stop the leak at once. To do this, you press your finger or the heel of your hand firmly against the nipple of the unoccupied breast and hold it there for the first minute or two of nursing; when you remove the finger, there will be no leaking.

You might tuck a gauze pad or clean folded hanky in each side of your bra. If you get the tingly, stinging sensation of the let-down, or feel the milk starting to leak, you can then fold your arms and press unobtrusively with the heel of your hand; or cup your chin in your hands and press against the breasts with your forearms, or some such maneuver. If a few drops do come out, the hanky or pad will absorb them. With a little experimentation, you can work out the ways of managing that will suit you best.

This might be a good place to suggest that if Christmas happens to come round while you're making starry-eyed plans for the arrival of the infant, and someone asks you for a gift suggestion for your husband, look innocent and say blandly, "White handkerchiefs." Your husband won't mind. Better some nice soft white hankies you can use than a hideous tie he can't. As we mentioned above, you will find that another item with tremendous possibilities in this respect is a clean diaper. Besides being useful to grab in a hurry to catch the overflow from the other breast when you start nursing, a clean diaper is just the thing to toss over your shoulder quickly to protect your clothes when you are holding the baby upright with his head on your shoulder—for burping purposes, or just because he seems to enjoy this position. Also good for flipping over the shoulder if nursing in a button-down-the-front dress in public.

Going Out? Take Baby Along

All babies, breastfed or bottle fed, need their mothers. But you don't have to be a stay-at-home with a breastfed baby. Baby can go right along with you almost everywhere you'd want to go. No new mother, for her own sake, ought to be out gadding much for a while, but when you're ready for a short trip for groceries, or a ride in the car to Grandma's, baby is an easy bundle to take along. And what better place to nurse him than in your car? Anyone for a drive-in movie?

It is possible to nurse inconspicuously almost anywhere, whether in your own home or that of a friend with others around. In the first place, there is nothing immodest about the partly bared breast of a nursing mother, and in most parts of the world no one gives such a sight a second thought. But of course we are living in *our* part of the world, and if your own feeling of modesty, or the feelings of those around you, should be offended, it's perfectly simple to conceal the whole operation. You will need only a minute or so of privacy to get the baby started nursing. Turning your back will do nicely; but if you feel awkward about it, you may prefer to slip into another room—the women's rest room, for example, in a public place. Those two-piece outfits we advised you to get will come in handy here. Sweaters can

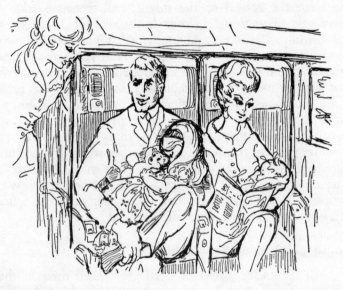

Is she or isn't she? Only baby knows for sure

be inconspicuously pulled up; the baby will cover your partly bare midriff, and no one will be the wiser. If you are wearing a blouse that buttons down the front, you can unbutton the bottom buttons, pull up the blouse a bit, and nurse the baby without embarrassment. The diaper or little blanket, as we stated, can be a casual cover up.

A photographer taking some pictures for a feature story about breastfeeding once asked Marian Tompson to pose holding her baby "just as if you were nursing him." But when Marian held the baby in the familiar position, he started nuzzling at her blouse in a frustrated sort of way. She excused herself for a minute, went into the next room and got the baby started nursing, then returned and posed obligingly for the pictures. The point of this story is that the photographer was completely amazed to learn later that he had gotten some real action pictures.

In other situations, other "cover-ups" can be used. On the beach, a large beach towel thrown casually over the shoulders and arms can serve as a kind of private tent for the nursing baby. And this doesn't look at all unusual either; people at the beach often protect themselves in this way from the sun or wind.

You will probably be able to work out plenty of casual methods for inconspicuous nursing to suit the places and people you are used to. Until you are very sure of yourself, though, you will probably feel happier about it if you try them out at home first, with your husband or a good friend as critic of the performance.

As you do become more sure of yourself, you may find the problem is not how to nurse inconspicuously, but how to tactfully discourage people who ask to "see the baby," completely unaware that he's busy filling his tummy. Gloria W., another League mother, asks, "What can I do about this short of hanging out a sign: MEALTIME—DO NOT DISTURB?" In this situation a sweet smile and finger to the lips implies that the baby is sleeping. If appropriate, you can whisper softly, "Later." Thus, you further the illusion by indicating that you have the kindly intention of displaying the child as soon as possible.

A practical hint on a good way to "tote" the baby when you are going somewhere and it isn't feasible to use your buggy or stroller is a baby carrier we suggested earlier (page 25).

If you *must* leave your tiny baby (and try not to any more than you have to), leave him with someone he is happy with when you're around. Here's where a teen-age brother or sister is wonderful, or a proud Grandma if she's been around the baby a lot. Daddy often fills the bill. Leave him well fed and contented. Don't rush—babies can sense when you are in a hurry to "get rid of them." When he's happy and settled, go off, do your bit of shopping, go to church, or take the older children to school. Don't be gone past his next feeding time, though, which means that for some time you won't leave him for longer than a couple of hours at a stretch.

Does that make you feel panicky and tied down? It shouldn't. You're a mother now, and you and your baby will both be happier if you are there when he needs you. Also, one of the big points of breastfeeding is that it is possible to take baby with you quite casually practically anywhere you might want to go. None of us are what you'd call the stay-at-home type, yet we manage. Mary White, who has traveled far and wide via plane, boat, and car during the last eighteen years (and nine children), has *never* left a nursing baby long enough to require a bottle. She has even been matron of honor at a wedding with her three-month-old baby held by the baby sitter, who came just for that purpose. Between church and reception, she slipped off, nursed the baby, and was back in the receiving line in time to shake a few hundred hands.

Some mothers feel that a baby isn't welcome at adult gatherings. The opposite is often true. Most people love to see babies, and there isn't a better "conversation piece" going. There's nothing like a baby to relieve tension or awkwardness.

After all, it never occurred to you to leave the baby behind when you were pregnant; it wasn't always exactly convenient, but one way or another, you managed. You can manage with your tiny baby now, too, because babies need to be with their mothers. The newer they are, the more they need them. Home is still best, though, most of the time, for both mother and baby. You are better able to relax in the old rocking chair in the old familiar surroundings than anywhere else. Even the fairly new baby seems happier amid the sight and sounds of home.

Very rarely, a situation might arise in which you *had* to be away from your tiny baby for longer than a few hours at a time. (Hospitalization is the only one we can think of offhand; but there might conceivably be others.) In that case, you'll find directions on pages 108-10 for hand-expressing, storing, and preparing breast milk to be given in a bottle. It isn't likely that you'll ever need to consult this; it's just there for the few people who *might* need it in unusual circumstances. Most of all, remember that baby needs someone he's familiar with, who you know will give him as much loving care as you would yourself, to be happy while you are gone.

Night Feedings

When your baby wakes at night, you need only tuck him into bed with you, start nursing him, and the two of you can drop off to sleep together. It's quite safe—we've all done it, and baby loves the warm closeness which usually helps

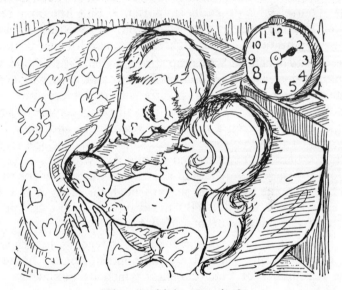

What could be simpler?

him drop off to sleep sooner than he might do otherwise. If you happen to wake again before morning, you can tuck him back in his crib if you want.

During the first two months, it is especially desirable for baby to wake for a feeding during the night; otherwise the mother's breasts might become uncomfortably full—a nuisance for her, and the baby might have trouble getting started nursing in the morning (see pages 61-62).

When Will He Start Sleeping Through the Night?

This is a matter of no real importance. Probably the reason the question ever assumed the proportions it has in the minds of some mothers is that, with the bottle-fed baby, it is inconvenient, and in winter chilly as well, to get up, warm a bottle, and sit up while you feed it to the baby. The nursing mother does not suffer such inconvenience. If she keeps the crib right near her bed, she has only to scoop the baby up in her arms, and she and the baby can lie back in bed snug and warm under the covers. So instead of fretting because Mrs. Brown's baby sleeps through the night and yours doesn't, ask yourself, "Is it really important? Isn't the important thing that my baby is content and happy because I am here to satisfy his needs day or night?"

As to when he will sleep through the night, it's impossible to say. Babies are human beings, and each and every human being in the world is different from every other. As adults we accept the fact that not all of us require exactly eight hours of sleep a day—some need more and some less. We understand that some people "simply can't eat breakfast," while others can't get started on the day without it. As we allow for these differences in adults, we must allow for them in babies. Some babies will sleep through the night at an early age, and some will not. (By the way, this is just as true of bottle-fed babies as of breastfed babies.)

If your baby is waking for a night feeding, he needs it, or else (especially with a baby six months or older) he needs the reassurance of your closeness which he gets when you hold him for his middle-of-the-night snack.

Still later, a toddler who wakes often at night may be bothered by teething. Even though he does not seem to be bothered during the day, perhaps the gums throb more at night when he is relaxed. Have you ever had a mild toothache that started throbbing madly just as you were dropping off to sleep? The toddler can't tell us about this; but, since waking up several times during the night is so common in children during their second year, we suspect that teeth might have something to do with it. Of course, many one-year-olds have funny eating habits and they may really wake up hungry. Whatever the reason, nursing does seem to soothe such a baby-child. (Which is he at this point? It's hard to say.) The milk that he gets from such a midnight snack won't be too significant nutritionally because your supply will have dwindled by this time as he is satisfying his hunger with other foods; but the nursing, coupled with your reassuring presence, does seem to soothe and quiet him, and that's the main thing.

If you think it might be hunger waking him, you might see to it that he gets a good bedtime snack and the equivalent of three or four square meals a day. Don't let him go thirsty either. Water or fruit juice, especially in warm weather, might be the answer. Overtiredness might be causing your baby to be wakeful. Check on the situation. Is he getting enough fresh air and exercise? Any tensions during the day? Frightening experiences? Enough loving? Enough freedom? If your answers to all these questions are satisfactory to you, and your toddler is *still* waking at night, blame it on teeth and remember that it will pass.

Twins—A Double Blessing

How do you manage with twins? "The rewards are great," says one mother of twins, "but during the first three months you won't have time to think about it."

The first question which seems to occur to the expectant mother of twins is often—"*Can* I nurse?" All of our doubly-blessed mothers agree that this is no problem. The more you nurse, the more your milk supply builds up. None of the mothers of twins we have known has had any difficulty supplying enough milk for two. The law of supply and demand seems to work just as well for "doubles" as for "singles." Lee M., whose ninth and tenth each weighed eight pounds at birth, still found no need to resort to supplementary bottles or to start solids earlier than usual.

Another mother of twins nursed them in the face of some rather determined opposition on the part of the hospital nurses, who told her that it was impossible to nurse two, gave them supplementary formula at first, against the mother's wishes and unbeknownst to the doctor, and brought bottles at each nursing period to make sure "*their*" babies got enough liquid. Luckily, the mother had the support and encouragement of her husband, her mother, and her grandmother, and with these reinforcements she stuck to her guns and nursed *her* babies.

Incidentally, she noticed that she had a terrific appetite and was unusually thirsty while nursing twins. She made a practice of eating an extra meal before going to bed. Other mothers of two could well follow her example in this, making sure that in the rush and excitement of twins their own nutritional requirements are plentifully taken into account.

In planning for two (and we hope you have prior notice so you *can* plan), take everything we have said and double it. In the twin household, cut your work to a minimum because sleep will be your problem, not milk supply. You can certainly build up an adequate supply of milk. However, your babies need the same relaxed loving attention that every baby deserves, and a tired mother is hard pressed to give this. If you possibly can, get yourself some help for the first few months. Your spare minutes should be spent resting and relaxing the way you like, and answering the needs of the other members of your family, not dusting, washing, or catching up on the unfinished work. You get extra help for your household work so you can manage and love babies.

Because twins usually come in smaller packages they need the protection of your breast milk even more than single babies. This thought seems to have encouraged several mothers to start nursing twins even when they had never nursed before. Edith H. successfully nursed two when she had never nursed her other children. Mary R. successfully breastfed twins after she had failed with her attempts at the previous six. "Can you imagine my finding the answer to relaxed mothering with my twins, when I never seemed able to nurse the other six?" is her comment.

Most of our twin-mothers prefer to nurse each of their babies separately. They thereby feel they are giving each one the time and attention that belongs to an infant. Separate feeding is *obligatory*, if the twins demand feeding at different times and raise a fuss when fed simultaneously. On the other hand, there might be times when it is easier to nurse them simultaneously, particularly during the early weeks or months when both tiny babies may wake up starving at the same time.

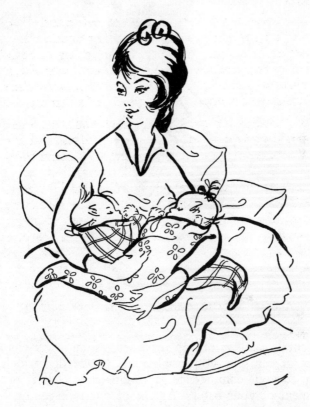

One convenient way to nurse your twins together

So much for some special hints for twin-mothers. We seem to have concentrated on the work involved and the need for a relaxed mother rather than highlighting the rewards of twin births. However, our files contain many glowing comments on the interesting adventure of nursing and raising two. With twins, your attention is focused on your babies in a special way. Just watching them, noticing their differences, their uneven growth pattern, their inherent tem-

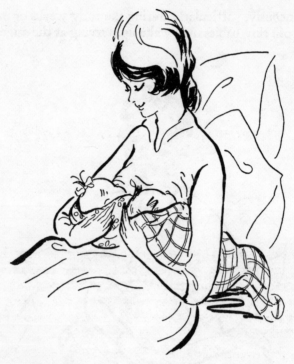

Another way to manage simultaneous nursing

peramental leanings, is an ever-interesting, ever-changing process. It can give you insights and knowledge which add greatly to your competence as a mother, as well as to your enjoyment of your babies. As one of our twin-mothers puts it, "I'm afraid having one baby will be rather dull, after watching two bloom and grow!"

Chapter 7

Special Circumstances

In this chapter, we are going to suggest how breast-feeding can be managed when there is some kind of special complication. In such situations you are not deciding all by yourself what should be done; your doctor makes the medical decisions, and when hospitalization is involved, hospital facilities and regulations must be considered too.

In any event, make sure your doctor knows that you want very much to breastfeed your baby, and that you are prepared to take some trouble to do so. His decisions about treatment are based on an evaluation of all the factors in a given situation; and one of the important factors is your own attitude. If he thinks you are lukewarm about breastfeeding, he may decide that it is best not to start or continue it under certain circumstances. On the other hand, if you are very much in earnest about nursing your baby, he may take this into consideration and go along with you. So be sure to let him know how you feel about it.

Many hospitals and doctors who know about La Leche League take advantage of our desire to cooperate in any way we can with a mother who is breastfeeding her baby under difficult circumstances. If your doctor is not familiar with the League, you can call this offer to his attention. Then, if he deems it advisable, he will get in touch with us.

The reason we especially urge breastfeeding in these situations is that it is even more important for a baby who runs into some complications at or shortly after birth to have the physical benefits of breast milk and the emotional benefits of the breastfeeding relationship as soon and as completely as he can.

Also, if you have already begun nursing your baby, switching him suddenly to a bottle plus an unknown mother-substitute can be a traumatic experience for him as well as for you. On your part, sudden weaning usually involves more or less painful engorgement of the breasts, which could lead in turn to a breast infection. On his part, the abrupt "desertion" by his mother, with all she means to him, has been known to upset a baby so much that if he is ill it slows down his recovery or, at the very least, leaves him confused and unhappy.

We are going to describe how such situations have been managed successfully, in the hope that this information may be of use to you and your doctor in the particular situation in which you find yourself.

WHEN BABY ARRIVES BY CAESAREAN SECTION

After a Caesarean you get off to a somewhat slower start, but there is usually no reason to anticipate any great difficulty with the breastfeeding. The baby may not be brought to you until the second day following delivery, and you will probably be in the hospital longer than usual, so unless you are in one of those wonderful hospitals that go all-out for nursing mothers, there may be a little delay in getting off on the right foot. But this kind of delivery does not affect your milk supply; all you need is a little patience. The same principles apply as with babies arriving the conventional way—no formula, and nursing every two or three hours, as with any new baby. Whatever the hospital situation, you will certainly be able to breastfeed the baby when you get home.

Because it will take a while for you to return to normal, physically, you will need more help with the house and the other children. This is true whether you are nursing the baby or not. Remember, the help you need is not with the new baby, but with other things. Be sure your helpers understand this. Handling the baby is *your* job; too many "mothers" will only upset him and make your job harder. You will find that nursing the baby is a most pleasant, restful occupation, and it is quite gratifying to know you are taking care of the most important job in the house with no effort at all.

Many mothers we have talked with or corresponded with have nursed with complete success following a Caesarean delivery, and you can surely do the same.

THE PREMATURE BABY

First of all, we should explain that there are many degrees of prematurity. At one end of the scale is the very tiny baby weighing only two pounds or so, in whom the wonderful modern techniques developed by dedicated doctors are barely able to keep the flickering flame of life alight. At the other end is the baby who, if he weighed just a few ounces more at birth, wouldn't be considered a premie at all.

In any case, if your baby is premature, this is a situation which has to be worked out in the way that is best for him, depending partly on the hospital facilities available. The very tiny premie may not be able to handle even breast milk for a while; he may be given a special solution by tube. When he is a little older, he may be fed breast milk, but should not yet be removed from the incubator. Still older, he may be put to the breast, but nurses so feebly that he requires much coaxing and patient handling.

The benefits of breast milk for the premie are well recognized by this time. In some cities, milk banks have been set up especially for the purpose of supplying it to such babies whose mothers don't know about giving their own milk.

So let your doctor know that you *do* want to breastfeed your premie as soon as you can. Your baby has been separated from you since birth, for even longer than usual; he will need not only the better nourishment but the warmth and closeness of the breastfeeding relationship even more than other babies. Keep in touch with what is being done for him, and keep hand-expressing your milk every two or three hours during the day (for method see page 108). If hand-expression proves difficult for you, the hospital may have an electric pump you can use, or you may be able to rent one when you get home. Hand pumps aren't as good.

Don't be concerned if you express only an ounce or so from both breasts at first. You will gradually work up to a better supply. Remember, too, that your baby is only able to take very small amounts at a time. Later, after the baby comes home, he will get more when he starts nursing.

What will happen to the milk you express? It will be used for your baby as soon as he can take it. (They may even give it to him with an eyedropper at first.) Until then, it might be used for other premies who for some reason are not so fortunate as to have a nursing mother; it might go direct to such a premie or be frozen and held in reserve in a milk bank. You will be discussing all this with your doctor and the hospital staff. They may have some special procedures for you to follow in handling the milk.

Dolores M. had to leave her two-and-a-quarter pound premature baby in the hospital incubator for two months. She hand-expressed faithfully several times a day and regularly sent the milk to the hospital. Joey took only about an ounce every three hours. By the end of two weeks, Dolores was regularly sending in sixteen ounces a day, the surplus being used for other premies. When she finally got him home, she had more milk than he needed at first, but the supply soon adjusted to his demand. Today Joey is a happy, healthy four-year-old. This was Dolores' eighth baby; while she was an old hand at breastfeeding, caring for a premie was a new experience for her.

Another mother, Eleanor H., delivered premature twin girls. Only one, Mary Jo, weighing less than two and one-half pounds, survived. Eleanor had two boys, six and seven, at the time, and had never successfully nursed either of them. But she was convinced that nursing was the best thing she could do for her baby in spite of being a high-strung person herself. She was most apprehensive about her ability to breastfeed; however, with the help of other nursing mothers, especially Dolores M., she was able to pump her milk and send it to the hospital.

While Dolores had always found hand-expression easier

and more efficient, Eleanor felt that she did much better with an electric pump during the time her baby was hospitalized. Little Mary Jo eventually came home and was happily breast-fed for over a year.

In some rare cases, the doctor-hospital setup may be such that your milk is not used while your premie is in the hospital. The baby will need it, though, when he gets home. So do keep up your supply by hand-expressing or pumping every day, at two- or three-hour intervals, for a total of about seven or eight times a day. You might freeze the milk (for procedures see page 109) for possible future use, either for your own baby or perhaps another, if there is a medical emergency and it becomes important to have breast milk quickly. Let your doctor know that you are doing this; he may like to know that there is frozen breast milk available, and he may be inclined to send the baby home a little sooner if he knows it will be getting breast milk there.

Certainly continual pumping or hand-expressing is time-consuming and calls for some sacrifice on your part, but when you weigh the benefits to the baby against the inconvenience to yourself and the rest of the family, there is not much question of what you will decide to do.

When you do get your premie home, be very patient with him. He may have considerable catching up to do, and he can use all the loving and mothering you can give him. He may have to be fed more often than other babies, and this will give you a good opportunity to cuddle him and baby him and let him know how much he is loved—a fact which his pro-longed hospital stay may have temporarily obscured for him.

IF THE MILK HAS DRIED UP

If, for whatever reason, the baby has not nursed for several days or even weeks, and your breasts are not producing milk, but you would like to start or resume breastfeeding, we have good news for you. It can be done. From time to time we hear from mothers who have taken the baby off the breast for one reason or another, usually because they had some kind of difficulty and thought they had to stop nursing. Then, discovering that this was not necessary, they wanted to resume nursing the baby again. While this is not as simple as nursing straight through from the beginning, or keeping up the milk supply by hand-expression if you are separated from the baby, it is not as difficult as you might think. A number of mothers who have asked us for help with this problem have come through with flying colors.

Probably one of the most dramatic experiences of this sort is that of Lorraine B., who, having tried unsuccessfully to nurse her first two babies, felt she was unable to breastfeed. Her next two babies were not nursed at all. Nor had her fifth baby, David, ever been at the breast. However, shortly after birth, he developed a severe diarrhea and eczema, and by the age of eleven weeks (*two and a half months*) he had reached a point where he could not tolerate any kind of formula or solid food. As a last resort, the doctor prescribed breast milk. Jean P., a nursing mother who lived in the vicinity, offered to nurse little David, and he immediately responded. After the first feeding of breast milk, the baby slept all night for the first time in his life, and thereafter his difficulties quickly cleared up. At this point the mother telephoned La Leche League for help. At our suggestion, she started nursing David for two minutes on each side about eight times a day, lengthening the sucking time as the nipples became less tender. She rocked and sang to the baby, and from time to time gave him a little breast milk donated by nursing mothers, giving it with an eyedropper while he was at her breast, to encourage him, before her milk came in. During the entire period Jean continued to nurse David each day. At the end of eight days Lorraine's milk began to come in—slowly at first, but gradually increasing until, at the end of a month and a half of concentrated effort, the baby was nursing completely at her breast, and the milk of the other nursing mother was no longer needed. Triumph!—made possible, we should add, not only by her own patient persistence, but by the unfailing support and encouragement of her husband.

So, if you haven't nursed your baby yet, or if you have stopped for some reason but want to start again, you *will* be able to do so—if you really want to do it and are willing to give yourself up to the time and effort it will take.

Just a word again here about dry-up medicine: in general, taking drying-up pills or shots will only partially or temporarily affect your milk supply. Stilbestrol principally relieves the engorgement which accompanies the first coming in of the milk. It will only reduce the milk supply in some cases. In any case, an actively sucking infant is capable of overcoming whatever depressive effects such medications may have.

How to Build Up Your Milk Supply

Even if you have taken dry-up medicine, all you need do is nurse the baby when he wants to be fed, bearing in mind that the breastfed baby needs to be nursed more often than the artificially imposed four-hour schedule. Every two to three hours is normal at first for the majority of babies (see page 63). The more often you nurse, the more quickly your supply of milk will increase. In between times, cuddle and hold the baby with complete abandon, and don't be afraid to put him to the breast for additional soothing, if this seems necessary, even though it isn't time for him to eat.

Naturally, the longer your baby has been bottle-fed, the more patience you will need to teach him to nurse at your breast. The sweetened formula (if that is what he was getting) and the relatively easy sucking needed to get the milk from the bottle have made him lazy and somewhat indifferent to nursing.

Essentially, here is the routine you will follow. At each feeding, first put the baby to breast. Coax him gently as you would a newborn, and if you have milk in your breasts, hand-expressing a bit in advance will help get the milk started for him. The taste of it might be all the baby needs to begin sucking. If so, wonderful. But if the baby is too hungry, or perhaps confused by this "new" routine, and refuses the breast, offer him a little of your milk (or that of a donor, if you need this kind of help to begin with) on a spoon or with an eyedropper. Prepare it just before you settle down to feed him and have it handy, so you won't have to be jumping up and down in the middle of a feed. After he has taken a half-ounce or so in this way, switch quietly back to the breast and coax him some more. Depending on how willing he is, and on whether or not you have milk to begin with, you will want to repeat this process once or twice at each feeding. Don't be discouraged if this takes some effort; persevere and, maybe not the first time, but soon, your baby will be nursing beautifully. Remember the experience of Lorraine B.

If the infant has been completely on formula for a considerable length of time, or if, because of lack of confidence or misinformation, you have been giving him more and more supplement, so that your own milk supply is *very* low, you will need to cut down gradually on the formula as you are building up your own milk supply. Here is the basic plan:

First Week.— Offer three-fourths of the usual formula (minus the sugar) and one-fourth added water (this is *besides* the water in the formula). Each time nurse the baby first—every two or three hours. Keep trying to get him to take the breast for at least a few minutes. His hunger will make him suck vigorously. Try for five minutes on each breast at each feeding, and before the week is out work up to ten minutes or longer.

*Second Week.—*Dilute formula still further to half formula (minus the sugar) and half water. Same procedure as above, only now you should nurse regularly ten minutes or longer on each side.

*Third Week.—*Baby will probably be taking well to the breast by now, and as soon as he does, the formula can be cut out entirely. Until then, limit formula to two ounces at each feeding, consisting of one part formula (minus the sugar) and two parts added water.

Of course, the younger the baby, the less formula he will have been taking and the less time the change-over will take. A baby only a week or two old may need only a few days or so to get back on the breast; the same holds true for an older baby who has been off the breast for only a week or so. Watch the baby, not the book, and don't feel bound to the three-week plan if your baby and you don't need that much time to make the switch.

It is most important, no matter what anyone tells you about the impossibility of getting back the milk supply, *that you believe in it yourself.* It *is* possible, and it has been done by many mothers whom we have helped. You have to really and truly want to accomplish it and be willing to devote the necessary effort to it. It does take a bit of doing—but it can be done.

IF YOU ARE ILL

For such minor ills as a cold or the flu you wouldn't even consider stopping nursing. The contagion is *not* transmitted through the milk. The baby has already been exposed to the germs causing your illness before you even knew you had them, and breastfeeding is probably the best protection against them. Also, a sudden change in method of feeding is hard on both of you. You need the extra rest afforded by breast-feeding, and baby still needs you. So keep nursing as usual, and don't worry about his catching your cold, or flu, or whatever. Very likely he won't get it. If he does, it will probably be mild.

In case of a more serious illness, or accident, you and your husband have to discuss the whole situation with your doctor and work out the plan that will be best for you and the baby. If you have to be hospitalized for a time you would need, as part of your care, to have your breasts pumped regularly, for your own comfort and welfare. Depending on the condition causing the separation, it may be possible to have this milk brought to your baby for bottle-feeding. If this is not possible, temporary arrangements might be made with another nursing mother either to send her milk to your baby or to nurse him herself. (If you don't know one, you might get in touch with La Leche League; see pages 151-155.)

Whatever arrangements you make for the time when you have to be separated from the baby, you will of course want to return home and to breastfeeding as soon as possible. In this case, arrangements for help in the home, and perhaps for your care as well, will need to be made, and continued as long as necessary. If the household responsibilities, and any special care you might be needing, are capably handled by others, your recovery would not be retarded but if anything speeded up by being reunited with baby. Nursing is "a drain on the mother" *only* if she is starving. Normally, the only thing the baby drains is the milk which was put there just for him. Your appetite takes care of the rest.

More than one mother we know had to be hospitalized when their babies were only a few weeks old. The doctors in these cases permitted them to bring their babies with them and keep them in their rooms, even though these hospitals did not have rooming-in arrangements. What wonderful doctors and hospitals!

IF YOUR NIPPLES GET SORE

Sore nipples aren't an illness, but they *can* be pretty uncomfortable. It's true that many times a little tenderness will clear up even if you do nothing at all about it, and some authorities advise this course. However, because you can't tell ahead of time whether the tenderness is going to go away or get worse, we have found it wise to give the nipples the kind of prenatal care described on pages 28-29. If you have followed this routine, you should experience little or no difficulty, no matter how vigorously your baby nurses. If your nipples *should* become tender in spite of this prenatal care (or if you have omitted it), we think it's best to start giving them some special attention before they become really sore, without waiting to find out if they are going to do so.

Actually, exposing the nipples to the air is one of the most effective ways you can toughen tender nipples. It's easiest to start this right after baby is born. Drop the trap door in your bra and leave it open as much as possible. A soft, loose blouse will help. If your outer clothing seems to rub on the exposed nipple, irritating it, you might try the suggestion one doctor made to a League mother, who used it quite successfully. She bought two tea strainers, removed the handles, and inserted one inside each cup of her bra. Thus, no clothing touched the nipples, and there was air circulating around them at all times. You might want to do this for several days, until the nipples heal.

Any mild ointment your doctor prescribes will probably be helpful. The ointment most popular with La Leche League mothers is pure lanolin. This was recommended to us by a psychologist-mother who has nursed four babies of her own. She tried using a number of different ointments and found that in each case the healing component was lanolin. She asked her druggist to sell her pure lanolin from his bulk supply. Although most ointments contain it, lanolin is not usually sold in its pure form because it is quite thick and sticky, and its odor, though not unpleasant, is not perfumed. The stickiness is actually an advantage for our purpose, because it stays on better. Lanolin is not harmful to baby; if applied sparingly, it is not necessary to remove it before nursing him. This is *not* true of all ointments, so if you are using another kind recommended by your doctor, better check with him about whether and how to remove it before nursing.

As we mentioned before, it has been our experience that alcohol, tincture of benzoin, and similar drying agents and soap tend to be irritating, so avoid using any of these things. Some mothers have had allergic reactions to detergent residues in their laundered bras, and have had good results from using disposable nursing pads or, more economically, disposable diapers cut into nine sections, with the plastic backing removed. Avoid plastic-coated pads in your bras; they can cause trouble, especially in hot weather, by holding in moisture and keeping out air; occasionally mothers have developed a rash from contact of the plastic with the skin.

If soreness persists even after the above suggestions have been tried, a sunlamp may be used. Mothers in tropical climates, whose breasts are customarily exposed to sun and air, don't seem to have sore nipples. Some doctors try to duplicate this by ultraviolet ray sunlamp on the breasts. An expensive lamp is not necessary; you can buy an ultraviolet bulb and put it in any lamp stand or socket. Sitting four feet from the lamp, expose yourself no more than one-half minute the first day, one minute the second and third days, two minutes the fourth and fifth days. If there is no indication of skin reddening by this time, you may increase to three minutes on the sixth day and maintain that level once a day until the soreness is gone. If you *do* notice a redness at two minutes, cut down to one minute and continue at that level for several days. Then try gradually increasing, one-half minute at a time, to see if you can tolerate a longer period. If not, keep it at the level that is best for you.

Be extremely careful always to protect your eyes with a towel or other cover while you are using the lamp; be careful about handling the bulb after use—it gets very hot; be careful not to get a sunburn from the lamp. It is imperative that you time yourself with a clock or watch.

Some mothers think that nursing less often—say every four hours, instead of two or three—will help sore nipples. The opposite is more often true. Easygoing, leisurely nursing every two or three hours is actually easier on nipples that are tender, because then the breasts don't become overfull, and the baby doesn't get so ravenously hungry that he nurses overvigorously.

You must remember, too, that there can be a relation between apprehension on the part of the mother and sore nipples. Slightly tender nipples may cause enough tension to hold back the let-down reflex. The delay in the milk may make the baby angry so that he pulls and tugs at the nipple, making it even sorer—and creating greater concern on your part. What can you do about this? You can hand-express a little milk to start the flow; and you can make a deliberate effort to relax before nursing. See suggestions on pages 77-78.

Some doctors recommend taking aspirin (but not oftener than every four hours) during the time your nipples may be painfully tender. *Consult your doctor in this matter.*

It also helps to change your position at each feeding, to put the greatest pressure in different places. Sit up for one feeding, lie down for the next.

During the time the nipples are quite sore, it may be necessary to limit the nursing time to ten minutes on each side. This will provide the baby with all the nourishment he needs. According to studies, he'll get nearly 90 per cent of the milk in the first seven minutes. However, this may not satisfy all of his *sucking* needs, especially if he has been in the habit of nursing for longer periods. A pacifier may be helpful here, but don't try to substitute the pacifier for mother. It probably won't work if you pop it in his mouth, put him down, and go off and leave him. Instead, continue to hold him at least as long as you would if he were nursing for the usual time. Then you will be satisfying both his sucking need and his need of you. The one-piece rubber pacifier is the safest. If he spits it out the first few times you offer it, don't give up. Coax him a bit, and chances are he'll take it. As soon as the nipples heal, go back to the full nursing period and discontinue the use of the pacifier. It may be difficult to establish a good natural nursing pattern if the baby relies on the pacifier for a considerable amount of sucking satisfaction. Limited use at this early age will not establish a habit or interfere with his oral development, but it's best to get him back to your breast for his sucking needs as soon as you can.

Some mothers have given up nursing because of sore nipples. This is unfortunate, because it isn't necessary. The nipples can be treated in the way we have described while you continue nursing, and the soreness will usually persist only for a few days. Only in very rare cases of *extremely* sore nipples, which might occur if there has been no preparation before the baby is born, and no treatment of beginning tenderness—only in such cases may it be necessary to discontinue breastfeeding, and then only temporarily. During this time the mother may have to hand-express her milk (see page 108) and give it to the baby in a bottle. As soon as the nipples respond to treatment, the baby can be put back on the breast.

Remember, though, that the proverbial ounce of prevention goes a long way in good nipple care and may save you considerable discomfort.

SORE BREAST
Plugged Duct?

It sometimes happens that a mother will notice a reddened area on the breast or near the nipple and/or a very tender spot, or a sore lump in the breast, sometimes accompanied by fever. The first thing to consider would be the possibility of a plugged milk duct. (Some doctors refer to this as "caked breast" or "milk fever" but stress that it is not a true breast infection since in most cases there are no bacteria present.) Frequently, this difficulty arises from inadequate emptying of some of the milk ducts. A too tight bra can cause a plugged milk duct if it presses on a milk gland and keeps the baby from getting all the milk out.

Sometimes all that is called for is the removal by soaking of the dried secretions that are covering the particular nipple openings. Also, be sure to let the baby nurse often, or a bit longer, especially if the breast is lumpy or you notice any hard areas. Hand-expressing the milk from the affected side after feedings would be helpful (see page 108). An ounce of prevention is particularly worthwhile here. Keeping the breast fairly empty and the milk flowing is the best way to improve the situation. Plugged milk ducts will soon be relieved by frequent nursing.

However, if you and your doctor are not sure whether the soreness is caused by a plugged duct or by the start of a breast infection, it won't hurt to follow the treatment described below.

Breast Infection

Breast infections if treated in time can usually be easily cured. If you should notice the soreness described above and it is accompanied by a fever, it is quite likely that you have picked up a breast infection. Your doctor may consider advising you to discontinue breastfeeding. Here, as in many other situations, your attitude will probably be a factor in his decision. If you can convince him that you feel very strongly about continuing, he will be more inclined to go along with you. While it previously was thought that a breast infection always meant that breastfeeding had to be discontinued, later studies have shown that continued nursing is not only possible but *advisable*. Abrupt termination of breastfeeding is a shock, emotional and physical, to both mother and child. The infection or plugged milk duct, whichever it might be, can become much worse if you do stop suddenly and allow the sore breast to become overfull. These studies also show that the baby is not harmed in any way by continuing to nurse. Doctors who care for many nursing mothers do not find it necessary to advise discontinuing the breastfeeding in this situation.

Our medical advisors give these three basic rules:

1. Apply HEAT.
2. Get plenty of REST.
3. KEEP THE BREAST FAIRLY EMPTY.

Get *lots* of rest (go to bed if possible), and apply heat to the affected area. If you can't stay in bed or on the sofa with a heating pad all the time, then try a small baby's hot water bottle, wrapped in a washcloth tucked inside your bra, to keep heat at the point of infection. *Be warned, though, not to let the resting go just because you're able to move about.* If the doctor prescribes medicine, take it and keep on nursing. Though some medicines pass through the milk— you can check with him about this—the effects are usually slight and are far outweighed by the advantages of breast-feeding. Until the infection clears up, let the baby nurse first on the sore breast at each feeding to be sure it will not become too full.

It might be that the location and nature of the infection are such that the doctor will want you to discontinue nursing from that breast temporarily; in that case you can keep nursing at the other breast for the time being, and hand-express and throw away the milk from the affected breast. You might suggest this possibility to him if he doesn't go along with your idea of continuing with nursing altogether.

Rarely, an infection may worsen and develop into an abscess. (This is much less likely to occur with the treatment mentioned above.) The doctor may decide to open and drain it. He might be willing to perform this small surgical procedure in his office, or even in your home. If he does prefer to hospitalize you for a few hours, you probably won't need to be separated from the baby for long. You would keep on nursing on the "good" side and hand-expressing on the affected side, while it's draining, to keep it empty. In a few days, you will probably be able to start nursing on that side again, just as if nothing happened.

We can speak from personal experience here, since this very thing happened to one of us. As in other cases we know of, the abscess healed completely, nursing at both breasts was resumed, and the mother nursed this baby, like the others, until he was ready to wean himself. Incidentally, she has since breastfed her next baby with nary a twinge, and no hint of trouble. So there is no reason to feel that you must never nurse again, either this baby or any others you might have.

IF BABY GETS SICK

Breastfed babies do get sick occasionally, just like everyone else; but rarely do they get seriously ill. Their colds are mild, their resistance is good, and the thing to remember is that the best way to care for the sick baby is to continue to breastfeed him, along with any other treatment or medication the doctor may prescribe. (The rare exception to this would be if the baby were not to be given any nourishment whatsoever.) One good reason for continuing to nurse your baby is that there is less danger of dehydration when a breastfed baby is sick and not eating well; you will find that, no matter how sick, your baby will nearly always nurse at least a little. Being at his mother's breast is such a comfort and soother that he will make regular efforts to suck. Usually the sick baby wants to nurse more frequently. This not only comforts him but supplies the extra liquid needed if he has a fever.

Remember, however, that your baby may have some difficulties nursing if a stuffed nose prevents him from breathing. If he cries while at the breast, it's not because he's rejecting you; he's just frustrated and needs some assistance. Check with your doctor. He may prescribe nose drops or have some other suggestion.

The recovery of a breastfed baby who has been ill is often quite remarkable. It is not unusual for him to maintain his weight even during a rather prolonged illness, and many of us have been quite surprised ourselves at the speed with which he can bounce back to normal.

Be sure that you *never* give your baby any kind of medicine without your doctor's specific instruction. This also applies to aspirin, which most of us take so much for granted that we hardly think of it as a medicine at all. It is an im-

portant fact that the child under three years of age cannot
handle aspirin well, and giving it to him indiscriminately can
result in serious reactions. So, if the little one is fussy (perhaps

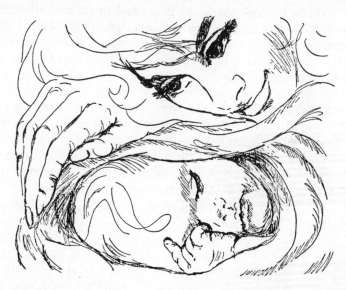

from teething?) *don't* give him aspirin without your doctor's
approval, and then use it only as directed, and for a limited
time, and be sure you are using the right tablet in the proper
dosage.

The Hospitalized Baby

If your baby is to be hospitalized for some reason, see
if you can arrange to be at the hospital with him so that you
can nurse him for at least some of the feedings. It has been
found that hospitalized babies and children generally recover
faster and the course of their convalescence is smoother when
their mothers are allowed to stay with them. Some hospitals
are very cooperative about this, allowing the mothers to
come and go with complete freedom and indeed encouraging
them to stay until baby is asleep for the night or even through
the night. Others view such a suggestion with much conster-
nation. It is interesting to note that the hospitals which ap-

prove and encourage this plan do so because they have tried it and found it most successful. Those against it have had little or no experience with this type of care.

When fifteen-month-old Brian had to enter the hospital for a major operation, his parents, our own Marian and Tommy Tompson, and their family doctor wisely chose a children's hospital which encouraged mother and baby togetherness. Here Brian and his mother roomed together day and night for all but two days of his twelve-day stay. During those two days in a special postoperative room she was still with him all day. Not only was recovery fast after surgery, but once home Brian exhibited almost none of the emotional reactions often seen in toddlers who have been hospitalized. He didn't cling to his mother, or cry if she left the room or house. He was also breastfed throughout this period.

If every wile and strategy have failed and you are not allowed to be at the hospital with the baby, express your milk regularly. Send it in to him (as you would with a premie—see page 109), so that it can be given to him in a bottle or by cup or spoon; or, if the doctor and the hospital do not see their way clear to using it for your baby, freeze it for possible future use. In any case, keep on hand-expressing (or pumping, if you prefer) to keep up the milk supply, so that you can put him back to breast immediately when he gets home.

Of course, through this whole difficult situation you will be conferring with your doctor, and he will help you work out the particular plan which will be best for your baby. He may have doubts that you will be able to keep up your milk supply; but if you convince him that you're in earnest and that you can do it, he will take this into consideration in deciding on the best course of action. One mother we know, whose baby had to be hospitalized for a whole month, persisted with expressing her milk even though she had three other small children to care for, and when the baby came home she was producing a quart of milk a day. So it can be done, if you have the love and determination to do it.

Remember, the hospitalized baby will have *greater* need of his mother's loving care. This is not the time to wean him.

No one really knows how much the baby misses his mother, or how terrified he can become at being kept in a strange place with strange people doing things to or for him. That is why breastfeeding is so especially wonderful for these babies.

THE RETARDED BABY

In past years, parents were strongly advised to place their newborn retarded baby in a home or institution where "special" care could be given. Now doctors are finding that your retarded baby needs the "very special" care which can be given best by you, his mother. Mongoloids, for example, do much better physically and mentally if kept in the warm, loving environment of their own home and family.

Along with this, of course, goes breastfeeding—an integral part of that very special kind of mothering which only you can give. Your retarded baby can be successfully breastfed with little more effort than any other baby. Some of these little ones do not have the strong urge to nurse and cannot show their feelings by crying energetically to tell you they are hungry. They are placid, contented, and may even happily go hungry unless you do a bit of clock-watching. But follow the usual two- to three-hour suggested schedule, and your little one will do very well. Some extra coaxing may be needed to get him started nursing, as his sucking instinct isn't very strong. But persevere, and know that you are doing the best thing for him.

You will gradually come to realize, too, that the rewards of caring for your retarded baby are many and perhaps unexpected. The extra feeling of affection and solicitude shown by his brothers and sisters, your own feeling of pride and confidence in being able to care for him yourself, are reflected in every aspect of your life. You are awakened even more fully to the needs of others; your endless patience and the extra time you devote to this baby are really worth while. You feel truly a mother in every sense of the word, and we want to reassure you that you can and should be just as much a mother to your retarded baby as to any child you have.

HOW TO EXPRESS AND STORE BREAST MILK

We are including here some special directions for the handling of breast milk when it is necessary to express and store it for various reasons. You won't need to bother reading these unless we have referred you to this section in discussing the handling of some special situation.

HAND-EXPRESSION

Wash your hands. Cup the breast in your hand, placing your thumb above and forefinger below the breast, on the edge of the dark area (areola), and simply squeeze them together. Don't slide the finger and thumb out toward the nipple. Don't worry if nothing comes out the first few times you try it; you'll get the knack soon. Rotate your hand slightly back and forth several times in order to reach all the milk ducts. The ducts radiate out from the nipple to the back of the breast where they widen to become the "storage places" for the milk. You may get only a tiny drop or so at first, but this is encouraging proof that the milk is there. *Persistence* and *confidence* are the key words here. After you have worked on one side for about three to five minutes, start expressing from the other breast, repeating the process described above. Then, do each side once more. This changing back and forth gives the milk more of a chance to come down the ducts, and you will be able to get a bit more each time.

USING AN ELECTRIC PUMP

If you are using an electric pump, first follow the directions for getting it started. These will be included with the pump when you get it. Then, as it starts working, do a little hand-expressing at the same time. This helps let-down the milk. An electric pump has a fine pulling or drawing action, but it does not imitate the action of a nursing baby, which combines sucking with a sort of biting, similar to the squeezing of the fingers in hand-expression. Every so often it helps to move the hand farther back on the breast, too, to work down the milk.

With the electric pump, as with hand-expression, it is better to go from breast to breast a couple of times, in order to get the most milk out that you can. In other words, pump on one side for five minutes, then go to the other breast for five minutes; then repeat the process once more.

A word of caution about using an electric pump. Since it has a pulling action, and a rather strong one, which may irritate the nipples, it is wise to limit the time at first to five minutes on each breast, and increase the time gradually. If your nipples begin to get sore or tender, reduce the time again.

TO EXPRESS MILK FOR THE PREMIE IN THE HOSPITAL

You will need:

1. A cup in which to hand-express the milk. Stainless steel is excellent; a glass or china teacup will do nicely. (If an electric pump is used, a container for this purpose is included with the pump.)

2. At least two glass or plastic jars or freezer containers, with tight covers, which can be sterilized. Small containers which will hold enough for one feeding are preferable.

Follow the instructions for hand-expression, or those for the electric pump if that is what you will use. Then pour the milk immediately into one of the glass or plastic jars, cover, and store in the freezer.

Repeat the pumping (or hand-expression) about every two hours, for a total of seven or eight times a day. Each time, pour the milk into the container in the freezer, using fresh containers as needed. As the days go by, you will find that you are gradually getting more and more milk each time you express it.

Do not handle the inside of either the freezer container or its top. It must be kept scrupulously clean. As for the cup into which you express the milk, wash it thoroughly, with hot water and soap, rinsing well with hot water, after each use. Store it in a safe place—the refrigerator is handy.

The hospital might want you to bring the milk in every day or every two days. In that case, it can easily be kept in the refrigerator, unfrozen.

If you want to freeze your milk for longer than a week or two, it *must* be quick-frozen and kept at zero temperature. (Note: unless your refrigerator has a dual-temp freezer section, it probably will not be that cold, and you must use a separate deep-freezer.) In the ordinary refrigerator ice-cube compartment, you may keep the frozen milk for up to two weeks.

TO EXPRESS MILK FOR ANOTHER BABY OR FOR A MILK BANK

In general, follow the directions for expressing and freezing given above, unless the milk bank has some other system of storing for you to follow. In that case, of course, do as they say. In this situation, it is presumed that you are now nursing your own baby as well, so you naturally consider his needs first. There are two ways you can arrange this: (1) Either nurse your baby according to his usual schedule (according to his needs, that is), and then hand-express or pump after each complete feeding. (2) Or, as some of us have done, if your baby is taking only one breast at a feeding (usually this would be a baby over three months of age), you can express the milk in the other breast after each nursing. If you are using an electric pump, you might find it easier and less time-consuming to nurse your baby on one side and pump on the other at the same time. This usually means that you will get more milk, because the nursing of the baby has a much stronger effect than a pump does on the let-down on both sides. It is one advantage of the electric pump that it does not require two hands to operate.

Remember, though, when the time comes that you are no longer planning to give your milk, to cut down gradually on the pumping, since you have built up a supply much greater than that which your baby needs, and the sudden drop in demand might cause engorgement, just as sudden weaning would. So taper off gradually, simply by pumping out some of the milk whenever your breasts feel overfull and uncomfortable.

TO EXPRESS MILK FOR YOUR BABY AT HOME

There may arise a time—rarely, we hope—when you find you simply have to leave your baby during one of his feeding times. In this case, since it's usually something special, and you will know about it in advance, you can plan accordingly. Starting twenty-four hours before you are going out, express your milk as above, after each nursing, and store it in the sterilized bottle you have placed in the refrigerator for such use. The amount of milk you will get in this length of time is usually just about right for one feeding. (If it doesn't look like quite enough, you can add to it an ounce or so of sterile water.)

If you are using milk that has been frozen, do not let it stand at room temperature to thaw. Instead, put the container under running water, first cold, then gradually getting warmer until the milk has liquefied, then heat in a pan of water on the stove.

See the section on going out (pages 79-83).

Chapter 8

The Father's Role

The Father in Relation to the Nursing Couple

Rare is the man who is not both pleased and proud when his wife nurses their baby. He realizes that this is the natural and womanly thing to do. But also rare is the man who fully realizes how much he can do to make breastfeeding a successful and happy experience.

After birth, the intimate relationship between mother and baby continues. They are still a unit. For some time, the baby's only need will be for the loving care of its mother. Recent psychiatric research has pointed up the far-reaching importance of the sense of security a baby develops from its earliest days if its needs are met by the mother promptly and consistently. But the man who fathered the baby, who was his wife's mainstay during pregnancy and her comfort during childbirth, should not now retire to the background. Because the mother must care for the baby, the father must care for both of them. Far from feeling shut out, he must realize that he is needed now as never before.

Father as Provider and Protector

The husband who hears the father's role described as that of provider and protector understands what it means to be a provider all right. But protector? From what must he protect his family? There are no wild animals at the cave opening!

First of all, he should protect the right of his baby to its mother's milk. A better food for babies than breast milk will not be discovered. Its myriad advantages have been pointed out previously. Suffice it to say that it is made-to-order by the same mother who did such a fine job of nourishing the baby before birth. Though there is now a swing back to breast-feeding, most babies are still bottle-fed. A woman may hes-

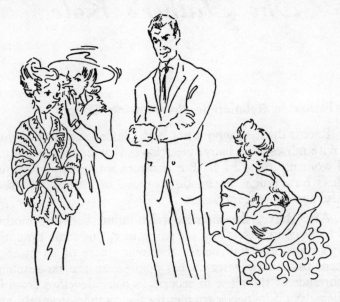

The protector

itate to be the only nursing mother on the block. She worries about what friends and relatives will think. But she is most sensitive to what her husband thinks. If she knows that she is more of a woman in her husband's eyes when she nurses the baby, the battle is half won. If he transmits to her the conviction that she can do what countless generations of women have done before her, she can hardly fail. Strangely enough, many women do not give the matter much thought during pregnancy. Often the encouragement of a clear-thinking husband is all that is needed to tip the scales in favor of breast-feeding. A woman who finds the whole idea of nursing a baby repulsive cannot, should not, be forced to breastfeed.

She should realize, however, that this is an abnormal attitude, indicative of underlying maladjustment.

Secondly, a husband has to protect his wife from the discouraging influence of well-intentioned but misinformed advisors. He is in an especially good position to defend their mutual decision to breastfeed when the criticism comes from *his* family; wives are extra-sensitive to remarks from this source.

When that fourth or fifth baby arrives, it is reasonable to expect everything to go smoothly. One of the rewards of a large family is the feeling of competence and confidence that the experienced mother has as she holds out her arms for her new baby. However, when the first baby comes, it is equally reasonable to expect things to go wrong. Not only does the baby have to make the adjustment from its insulated and effortless intrauterine existence to a life of heat, cold, noise, eating, and breathing, but the wife-become-mother is also going through a difficult transition period. At this point she is only a novice and it takes very little to magnify her doubts as to her own ability.

Her husband should dispel her doubts; not introduce new ones. The baby cries, her breasts seem empty, someone remarks, "You can't just let the child STARVE!" and she runs for a bottle. Here, in her mad leap from the frying pan into the fire (for bottle feeding brings problems of its own), is where hubby should catch her. He will reassure her, steady her, remind her that babies cry for reasons other than hunger.

Of great help to the mother at such a time is a talk with or a phone call to another woman who has been through the same thing herself. There is a better solution to the above dilemma than mixing up a batch of formula. The mother can just relax with a snack, something to drink, and a book, and let the baby nurse as long as he likes. More milk will be along and baby may surprise everyone by sleeping for five hours when he finally pops off. He just had an extra-fussy spell and needed some extra loving for a while.

The most important thing she must do, and the hardest, is to learn to have faith in herself as a mother. There is no substitute for time and experience. It is only these that transform the unsure mother of the two-week-old into the self-confident mother of the six-month-old. After a birth, as after a marriage or a death, there is a period of readjustment during which "business as usual" should not be attempted or expected. During this time there should be a reorientation on the part of both parents away from some of the more couple-centered pursuits of the past toward family-centered living.

Finally, a nursing mother may also need to be protected from herself. Some women, in their eagerness to be good wives and mothers, to do all things well, to keep the house immaculate, to be well informed, to take part in community affairs, to look lovely for their husbands, simply run themselves ragged. They may become so bogged down in the many details they must attend to that they lose sight of their goal. They need to be reminded to sit down and eat a good meal. They need to be encouraged (or even told) to rest occasionally. They may grumble that they "ought to" be doing such and such but will later proudly "complain" to friends that "Joe insisted that I lie down for awhile." In short, they need their man to help them keep the right perspective—to put first things first—to reassure them that a relaxed and cheerful wife and healthy, happy children are greater values than sparkling windows or powdered noses.

Father as Helpmate

There are times when a woman may find that just taking care of the essentials is too much. When she has just returned from the hospital with a new baby, for example; or when an ill or fussy child results in her putting in more time "on the job" in two or three days than her husband puts in in a week. At such times, the considerate husband sees that she gets some assistance. Hired help is nice, if you can afford it (and if you don't mind the lack of privacy). Women relatives are nice, if you've had the foresight to acquire some (and if they don't take over the house and the baby). Lacking these, it is desirable that hubby, as the second adult in the family, volunteer to lend a hand.

Unfortunately, however, there has been a good deal

written lately ruling "woman's work" or acting as a "substitute mother" out of bounds to the man who values his masculinity. Much confusion has taken place in many modern homes in the roles of husband and wife, the experts say. Often both are wage earners, both care for the children, both do the housework—and sometimes the woman is definitely the boss with father relegated to the role of "mother's little helper." As a result of this blurring of functions, "a child doesn't have a clear father or mother image. No wonder so many boys and girls are mixed up about their roles in later life."

> The star of the television program, "Father Knows Best," tells what happened when Father was in the kitchen and, instead of just standing around, helped his wife dry the dishes. "We received a flood of mail. Many of the letters protested that we were trying to make Father into Mother and said that dish-drying isn't man's work. . . . This comment was a huge surprise to me, because nowadays most families, like Jim Anderson's, do not have household help and fathers pitch in with the chores. Jim just did what came naturally."

Perhaps we might take our cue from that—doing what comes naturally—without worrying too much about losing our masculinity on the one hand or our women's rights on the other. We are all in favor of manly men. And La Leche League was formed for no other purpose than to help women be more womanly. As you might guess, we're going to urge breastfeeding in order to help keep these father and mother images clear! Let's see the men take *that* over.

As long as women continue to bear babies and to nurse them, there is not much danger that the roles of mothers and fathers will become badly confused. While the pregnant or nursing mother, of necessity, stays at home, the father, of necessity, will go out and make a living. The wifely duties will consist of baby and child care, cooking, washing, ironing, and the many tasks usually associated with homemaking. During his "at home" hours, the man's greater brawn makes him a natural for carpentry, housepainting, putting up storm windows, fixing the plumbing, etc. Thus, there is, *on the whole*, a natural division of labor within the family.

The fact that certain duties are ordinarily performed by father or mother does not mean that under some circumstances they cannot be performed by the other. If a husband and wife like to talk over the dishes, or work together in the yard, hurrah for them! When there are several children, if they don't find companionship *doing* something, they may not find it. If one spouse is temporarily overburdened, love and reason impel the other to ease that burden. A woman does not lose her femininity if she helps her husband with work he brings home from the office. If a wife has been up much of the night, a husband grows in stature *as a man* when he has the thoughtfulness and foresightedness to let her nap with the baby while he takes the older children for a walk. An overtired woman cannot be a good wife or mother, nursing or otherwise.

We would agree with the psychologist who says, "A wife who shifts her unpleasant household chores to her husband is downgrading her own activities in her children's eyes." (She might ask herself if there isn't something wrong with her attitude if she regularly finds the duties of motherhood unpleasant.) We would say, in addition, that a husband who wouldn't be caught dead with a dish towel in his hand is also downgrading his wife's activities in the children's eyes. As one man put it, "I think that more important than what a father *does* around the house is *what he is*. The authoritative, masculine man knows his dignity and stature are not in jeopardy when he performs a kitchen chore."

Father as Companion

Substituting for his wife in child care may be an important function of the husband at times but it becomes less necessary as time passes. The care of older children can be more easily systematized and the children themselves can help with the household chores. But there is a husbandly function which will never be outgrown—the reason why he married in the first place—that of being a companion to his wife.

A woman who has been in the house with small children all day needs adult companionship, especially that of her husband. She likes to hear what is going on "in the world" and appreciates an occasional glimpse of it herself. Though woman's place may be in the home, so, outside of working hours, is man's. They both need and profit from outside interests but their first duty is to their family. Family activities and outings are wholesome and to be encouraged. Of course, it is not feasible or desirable to do everything "as a family" —we need aloneness as well as togetherness—but the time spent alone should enrich our family life, not impoverish it. There is no better way to abdicate one's position as head of the family than by never being around. Just and prudent authority cannot be wielded by absentee ballot, as it were.

This, then, is the kind of man the family needs: a good provider so the mother may devote herself to the needs of the children without distracting worries; a protector who will shield her from the doubting Thomases by having confidence that God knew what he was doing when he sent milk along with the baby; a helpmate lest the burdens of motherhood make her forget that children are a blessing; a companion because the joys of parenthood are meant to be shared.

This kind of husband makes for a happy and secure wife. A happy and secure wife makes for happy and secure children. The sum total is a happy family. Never underestimate the power of a man!

Chapter 9

Gradually, and With Love

We mothers want, perhaps more than anything else, to have the wisdom to guide our child's growth so that his personality comes to fruition unstunted and undistorted. We want him to become an independent, mature, loving person with his talents and abilities developed to their fullest.

We know that our first job is to meet his physical and emotional needs as fully as we can, so that a secure foundation is laid for his advance to maturity. We know that by breastfeeding him we are getting him off to the right start, and that the breastfeeding relationship itself makes us more sensitive to all his needs and quicker and surer in devising ways of meeting them.

As he grows, his needs change, and we must progressively let go of him as he assumes the direction of his own life. This process will not be complete until he is fully grown, but it does start now, in babyhood. This book, therefore, would be incomplete if we did not analyze a bit these beginnings of independence and our role in fostering them.

The biggest change with which we are concerned in infancy is the transition from nursing to eating adult foods. The other dramatic changes—growing in stature, walking, talking—go on more or less automatically; but we mothers do have a great deal to do with what and how the child is fed, and it is our responsibility to learn the best ways of managing this. Not that it is such a big chore—it is actually quite easy and fun, too, if done at the right time.

Most of this chapter, then, will be concerned with when

and how to introduce foods other than breast milk, and when and how breastfeeding will be discontinued. We will then look ahead a little and indicate how the same philosophy which guides us in these matters, expressed in the title of this chapter, applies also to some of the other events of early childhood.

INTRODUCING OTHER FOODS

First, a word about vitamin supplements. This, of course, is up to your doctor. Important medical authorities believe, with good reason, that if the nursing mother gets an adequate supply of vitamins, the milk will have an adequate supply of vitamins, in just the proper proportions. So your physician may prefer to give *you* the vitamin supplements, especially if you suggest it. As you perhaps may realize, vitamin supplements for babies got their impetus as a supplement to formula feeding.

Other Foods—When

Hand-in-hand with bottle feeding of babies, the fashion of starting to feed solids earlier and earlier developed and took hold in this country. One of the factors in this, as Dr. Spock and others have pointed out, is a spirit of rivalry and competition among mothers (and sometimes their doctors). Some mothers feel that it reflects great credit on them if their children do things *earlier* than their neighbor's children; and for many, during infancy, there is little to brag about but weight gain. They also earnestly try to get the children to walk, to talk, and go to the toilet as soon as possible; and if they could figure out a way to make them teethe earlier, they would probably do that, too.

The whole thing is ridiculous, of course; by and large, babies should develop at the pace Nature intended. If they are pushed too hard, or made to feel unloved because they are not performing as their mother wants them to, they may become tense, unhappy persons in the process, and in the long run the mother may pay dearly in anxiety and sorrow for her ambition to have *her* child do things earlier than others.

Today medical scientists are talking about *excessive* intake as well as *deficient* intake. They find that infants can be over-fed as well as underfed. Overfeeding can result from the premature introduction of solid foods. Breast milk, on the other hand, gives the best assurance of proper nourishment because it is Nature's complete food for your baby. It is the perfect food until about the middle of the first year after birth, and therefore there is usually no reason for adding any foods to the breastfed baby's diet in the early months.

There are at least two very good additional reasons for waiting.

First, you want to maintain your milk supply, and the more solids the baby takes, the less milk he will want; the less he takes from the breast, the less milk there will be. In other words, what you are doing is substituting an inferior food for a superior food. It is the mother who starts solids at around one month who complains that her milk is gone by the time the baby is five or six months old.

The second reason for waiting is that the younger the baby, the more likely it is that any foods other than breast milk will cause food allergies. No one food will *necessarily* do this; but you can't tell until you try. Cow's milk, used in most formulas, is the most common allergen there is. Many other foods as well may cause an unpleasant reaction in a two-month-old, but be readily assimilated by the same child by the time he is six or seven months old. It seems both the kindly and the wise course to give the baby the benefit of a few extra months of the food that Nature has devoted millions of years to perfecting for him, until his immature digestive system grows up to the point where it can utilize other foods without upsets.

At about the middle of his first year, or shortly thereafter, the supply of iron with which the full-term, healthy baby was born begins to give out; breast milk is no longer a complete food for him, though it is still a valuable part of his diet; and at this point, when he is ready for it and begins to need it, you start adding solid food. (In certain specific cases, a doctor might have a reason for starting solids earlier.)

The increases in appetite which occurred probably at

about six weeks and three months (see pages 73-74) were met merely by stepping up the breastfeeding to increase the supply of breast milk; the baby was not ready, physiologically or emotionally, to start solid foods then. In the middle of his first year, however, he will probably have started to teethe, and his natural urge to chew and bite is developing. His digestive system, also, is now ready to handle new foods. When his needs, capacities, and abilities make it logical, we begin to introduce them.

Your baby will probably let you know when he is ready; watch him, not the calendar. If he suddenly increases his demand to be fed some time around six months of age, and this increased demand continues for four or five days in spite of more frequent nursings, you can assume the time has come to start him on solids. If he is much younger than this, however, don't get excited at these first signs and rush the start of solids, because the demand might be due to other causes. A cold coming on might make him want the solace of nursing oftener. Or stepped-up activity on your part may have made you rushed and tense, and that may be bothering him. If he is fussy for some reason other than hunger, he will have enough to cope with without introducing an additional complication into his life. So play it safe and go along with his increased demands at the breast for a few days to make sure it is hunger that is responsible.

Other Foods—How

When you do start solid foods, you'll probably find that your first few attempts to spoon-feed your baby will be a bit clumsy. It will help if you remember that up to this time he has been used to sucking only. This involves pressing his tongue firmly on the underside of your nipple so that the upper side is against the roof of his mouth. The sensation produced as he tries to treat a cold, hard spoon the same way must be somewhat disconcerting to him. It is a good idea to nurse the baby before giving him his solids until he is eight or nine months old. First, this will keep up your milk supply and assure the baby's getting the best food first. Second, if he's ravenously hungry, he will be in no mood to try out something new. Take the edge off his appetite first and he'll be more willing to go along with you.

By the time he is six months old or so, baby's mouth and tongue are ready for the new skills, but he still has to learn them. Use a small spoon and, at the beginning, place just a small amount of food on the tip of it. These first feedings of solid food usually go more smoothly if you hold him in your lap, tilting him back slightly as you touch the spoon to his lips. With practice and patience on your part, he will catch on readily. Keep in mind that these first few attempts are merely to introduce the idea of solids to him, not to try to fill him up.

Many babies are ready for a high chair around six months and can handle finger foods fairly well—they just *naturally* put everything into their mouths. If you have an independent baby who balks at spoon-feeding, provide him with plenty of finger food instead, and by the time he's a year old he will probably be spoon-feeding himself beautifully.

New foods should be introduced one at a time. This means a single food, not a mixed food like stew or soup or even a mixed-grain cereal. The reason for this precaution is that although the baby at this age is not nearly so likely to have an allergic reaction as a younger child, it is still possible. If you are introducing foods one at a time, and he should develop a rash or a sore bottom, you will know which food has caused it and can eliminate it temporarily.

It's a good plan to allow four or five days or more between each new food introduced. There is no advantage to be gained by striving for a wide variety of foods in the shortest time possible. Rather it is good for the baby to be given the opportunity to experience each new food thoroughly before he goes on to another. Start with about a quarter-teaspoon of a new food. Increase it little by little until at the end of a week he is getting as much as he wants. He will probably let you know when he has had enough by turning his head away, clamping his mouth shut, spitting the food back out, or some such unmistakable gesture. Take his word for it. Don't start feeding problems now or ever by coaxing, pushing, or forcing. Give him only as much as he wants, not what you think he should have.

Once a food has been started, it should not be stopped completely for any length of time. For example, if the baby has had cereal several times and then you forget to buy it for several weeks or change to a different kind, it is possible for him to develop an allergic reaction on its reintroduction after this lapse of time. So, once a new food has been started, see that it becomes part of the baby's newly varied diet even if it is only a taste of it about once a week thereafter. This precaution should be kept up during baby's first year.

Other Foods—What

Most of us find it unnecessary to use the commercial baby foods at all. They are relatively expensive, and some varieties contain undesirable fillers such as sugar, and preservatives. If you do use jar foods, read the labels. Sometimes a doctor may recommend these rather than run the risk of a possible poor diet due to a mother's ignorance of proper food values. For instance, if a baby would be fed from the table a diet consisting mainly of starchy and sugary or highly spiced foods, such as spaghetti, noodles, white bread, and sweets, then certainly such a baby would be better off with a variety of strained jar foods. However, if you understand good nutrition, and your family's eating habits are pretty good, then the food from your table will probably be fine for your baby, too. This also makes the transition to family meals easier. (See Chapter 3.)

Some of us do use the baby meats to introduce this food to the baby until he is taking it fairly well. Then we switch to table meat. In buying these strained meats, we take care to get the same kinds of meat we serve the family; there is no point in getting the baby used to canned veal, or pork, or turkey, unless these are meats you serve frequently. Mothers with blenders would have no need to buy specially prepared baby meats.

Your doctor and your book on general baby care (Newton or another—see Booklist, page 144) will give you detailed information on what foods to introduce in what order; but for your convenience we'll include here the order which we have found works well for most people.

1. *Mashed Ripe Banana.*—This is a good first food with which to introduce babies to solids. It is a good natural food and contains more food value than the cereals. Babies usually love its smooth consistency when mashed with a little water. Very soon you can offer the baby a whole piece of banana to handle himself, thus quickly eliminating one mashed food as well as pleasing the baby, who likes to feed himself.

2. *Meat.*—This is introduced early among solid foods because of its high iron content. Use the strained meats for a month or so or your own table meat which you have prepared in your blender. Meat can be temporarily added to the mashed banana if the baby has difficulty accepting it. Later, when the baby is eating it regularly, switch to meat from the table. It is not difficult to reduce table meats to a consistency right for baby eating. The roasts and chops are not handled too easily at first, but chopped beef or stew meats, or tender pieces of chicken, can easily be mashed with a fork and moistened with the meat juices, breast milk, or warm water. When the baby has had a week on one meat, try handing him a good-sized bone with a few fragments of meat still on it. (A chicken leg bone is usually a good size for a starter—big enough to handle and too big to swallow.) Chances are he will chomp away on it with great relish, and it will help with his teething and muscular coordination too.

It's a good plan to allow about a week between each new variety. A good method of making sure you have the kind of meat your baby can handle is to keep individual portions of chopped beef, ground heart, or hamburger wrapped and frozen. When you have meat at the table that might be too difficult for baby, put the chopped meat into a saucepan over low heat, tightly covered or still in its aluminum-foil wrapper. The moisture from the frozen meat will steam it nicely in a few minutes.

Individual portions of liver, frozen as soon as purchased, are handy to prepare for baby in this way. They also make a good snack for the hungry toddler (or anyone else, for that matter), thawed, cut into finger-sized pieces, dredged with flour, and quickly sauteed in a little oil or bacon fat. When baby is older, all-beef frankfurters boiled for ten minutes make fine finger foods.

Egg yolk can be substituted for meat as the second food to be introduced. However, eggs seem to be one of the more common causes of allergies, and for this reason most of us wait until baby is about a year old before introducing them. The egg should be prepared as follows: hard cook the egg in water by cooking it below the boiling point—simmering—for twenty to thirty minutes. Feed baby only the yolk, mashed and moistened to suit. As with all other new foods, start with no more than a quarter-teaspoon and increase gradually, a quarter-teaspoon at a time. (Be especially careful to proceed slowly when introducing this food early.)

3. *Whole-Wheat Bread or Whole-Grain Cereals.*—Dried or toasted slices of whole-wheat bread cut into finger-sized pieces that baby can hold are good food for him and handy to offer him, perhaps between meals or while you are preparing his meal. At first more bread may land on the floor than in his mouth, but he'll catch on gradually, and there's no rush about it. If you regularly serve a cooked whole-grain cereal to your family, you might want to introduce this; but be sure there is no sugar or other sweetening added. Moisten with water or breast milk, not cow's milk, since this has not been introduced if you are following this plan. Baby cereals do not have quite as much food value as the whole-grain cereals and are an additional expense. If the whole-wheat bread is well liked, you don't have to bother with cereal at all unless it is convenient.

4. *Potato.*—Baked sweet potato is best, but baked white is also good. The sweet variety has not only maximum food value but a very smooth consistency when moistened with water, or perhaps with some of the strained meat. Babies love it!

5. *Fresh Fruits.*—Scrape some raw apple with a spoon and put a little of it in the baby's mouth. Soon he can have a little mound of it on his high-chair tray to experiment with, and it won't be long before you hand him a piece of ripe peeled apple, pear, or peach to munch on enjoyably. As he gets

older, other fresh fruits in season may be offered, but with caution. Berries have seeds which babies are not old enough to handle, and they may also cause a rash when introduced at an early age. Citrus fruits are a common cause of allergy when given early in infancy, and the baby should be introduced to citrus fruit juices only after dilution with two parts of water. This dilution can gradually be decreased. Avoid canned or jar fruits if possible. They contain sugar, which is not good nutrition for the baby, and they have less food value than the fresh variety. On the other hand, canned fruits with the syrup drained off, or strained jar fruits, are better than no fruit at all. Unsweetened canned fruit juices, such as apple juice, can also be added.

6. *Vegetables.*—Finely grated carrot mixed with raw apple goes down very easily; or grated carrot may be offered alone or mixed with some of the other foods the baby is getting. Cooked vegetables may be offered from your table (one at a time as you start any new food). Raw vegetables have more food value, but for the new eater most raw vegetables are too stringy and generally hard for the baby to chew and digest. Don't overlook root vegetables. Cooked beets and squash are usually quite acceptable to little ones.

7. *Whole Milk.*—You don't have to be in a rush about this, because your baby will still be nursing. But at about seven or eight months, you can start offering him milk *from a cup* once or twice a day—at mealtime or in between, whichever suits you best. Don't rush the drinking from a cup. For some time most of it will go down the chin. A tip on getting the baby started with a cup comes from Betty Wagner, and we find it works beautifully: let him drink through a short straw. The sucking comes easy for him, and it's lots neater too—no drips or dribbles. Pretty soon he'll catch on to the conventional way of drinking.

Remember, though, that milk is essentially an infant food. If your baby doesn't take to cow's milk, forget it. He'll get his nourishment from other sources and from foods cooked with milk. Furthermore, milk in large doses can displace more important foods by lessening the child's appetite for them. Because milk lacks iron, and the infant's storage of iron runs out after about six months, the child whose preference for milk cuts down on his solids may end up pale, pasty-faced, and anemic. (This condition is known as milk anemia.)

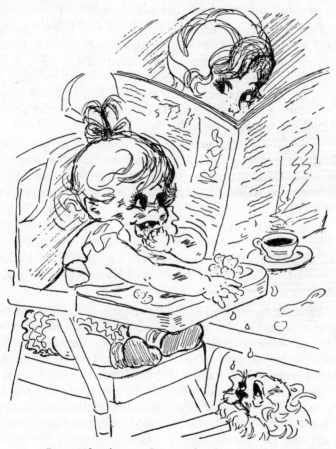

Finger foods are fun—and educational too

His beverages then should consist mainly of milk, water, soups or any unsweetened fruit or vegetable juice (check the label on the juice can). No soft drinks, please; carbonated or uncarbonated, these are heavy on sugar and sometimes caffeine and are stimulants lacking in anything worthwhile.

As to other foods, now that milk is introduced you can

slip butter in almost anywhere along the line. Do use it sparingly at the beginning and don't rush it; baby will enjoy his bread without butter, and until he gets a bit older it will be much less messy if he eats it dry. Cottage cheese can be started here—a good protein food and bland, too.

Fish is another excellent protein food. It isn't usually started as soon as meat or eggs, because it is not as rich in iron, the essential early addition to the breastfed baby's diet. But it is entirely suitable for him, and rich in other valuable nutrients, so if your family menu includes fish frequently, you can introduce baby to it too. Wait a while with the smoked and pickled varieties, though.

Hold off on condiments—catsup, mustard, pepper, horseradish, and so on—until he begins to demand what you have; then allow them sparingly. You'll find that for some time he will settle for a lot of fanfare and a minute speck of the condiment.

Skip sweetened desserts such as puddings, cakes, and cookies. Pass up the teething biscuits, too. These are sweetened, and he doesn't need them. He can teethe very nicely on crusts of whole-wheat bread, a chicken leg bone, a stalk of celery, or a raw carrot.

When baby has had a variety of each of the above foods, you can consider him well started on solids, and you will no longer have to think too much about introducing new foods. The whole process may take about three to six months, depending upon how eagerly the baby takes to solids. Notice that from the beginning, if you follow these suggestions, baby is eating as a full-fledged member of the family, from the table. You have given him good nourishment, avoided the expense of special baby foods; and there is no painful transition from strained foods to chopped foods. Merely moisten the food more freely for the first month or so, and gradually get it to a consistency that is not much different from the way the rest of the family has it.

You'll find that with finger foods it works well to give them to him on the high-chair tray, a piece at a time. When you are giving him softer foods with a spoon, and he wants to grab the spoon, the time-honored procedure is to give him a spoon too, and (eventually) the dish of food. You may be surprised at how quickly he can manage not only his own finger foods but his own spoon-fed foods as well. You'll save some messes and make the learning process easier for him if you have only one thing at a time on the tray—*one* piece of the finger food, later *one* unbreakable dish with a not-too-large serving of *one* food, and (not at the same time) a small unbreakable cup half-full of milk or juice. Keep servings small. Later on give him small finger foods like cooked peas. They will help him gain finger control and coordination.

Give him more of any food as he indicates he wants more. When he doesn't want more, stop. Baby's appetite is variable from meal to meal and from week to week. *Don't ever coax, wheedle, cajole, or force him to eat.* If he doesn't want to eat a certain food, try something else. Babies sometimes go on food "jags," eating practically nothing but meat or fruit or cereal for days at a time. Then suddenly they switch to something else. Go along with this, by all means. Babies who are allowed free choice of good, nutritious foods will always balance their own diets.

WEANING THE BABY

When shall I wean my baby? How shall I go about it? How long will it take?

Often mothers worry about this matter when their infant is only a few weeks old. Now, why on earth does this begin worrying them so soon? No doubt there are many reasons, but we suspect that not least among them is the fact that our society *expects* babies to be weaned early. A newborn at the breast is sometimes accepted in our American culture; an older baby, a toddler—never. This is true even though it is a common sight to see a two- or three-year old with a bottle. So, eager for social approval for ourselves and our children, we are uneasy about the thought that our babies might still be nursing after this accepted period.

Will you take another look at this attitude with us? We are going to assume that you agree with us that our norm for judging what we should do is what is best for our babies

—not what others think we should do. That being the case, this is how we look at it.

The breastfeeding mother and her baby build up a relationship based on their mutual needs, and the relationship changes gradually as the needs change. One of the most urgent needs of the *tiny* baby is for food, preferably milk, and during this period of infancy the mother's physical need is to be relieved of the milk that fills her breasts for the sake of the baby. However, mother and baby depend upon each other for many other things: the mother needs to give affection, the baby to receive it; the baby needs to hear his mother's voice, to feel the warm comfort of her body, and to be held; the mother has a strong desire to be truly needed by the tiny one dependent on her.

If we consider nursing only as a means of nourishing the infant, then we can readily see why it might be feasible to bring nursing to an end at an early date. There would be no reason why this date could not be as early as the baby could handle a variety of solid foods and milk from a cup—at whatever age that might be. But if we view the nursing experience as a whole, if we see this important, intimate relationship as a vital part of motherhood, meeting the total psychosomatic needs of the baby, then it is hard to understand why we should set a specific time when this relationship *must* be ended.

It is true that some doctors, nurses, and others who are strongly in favor of breastfeeding, up to a point, nonetheless advocate a definite age for weaning. On the other hand, many doctors, psychologists, social anthropologists, and other scientific folk (as well as mothers, in terms of their natural intuition), are equally outspoken in advocating a more relaxed attitude toward weaning the baby. They point out that in cultures where children are allowed to continue nursing quite freely as long as they like, the children in general are well-adjusted, gentle, agreeable persons when they grow up. To our way of thinking, the reasons offered by the first group for weaning at a certain age are not valid. The most common reason given is a fear that prolonged nursing will prolong the baby's dependence. The fastest road to independence, however, is traveled by the child who develops security during his dependent years—who can count on his mother's taking care of his needs. Among our children and those of many other mothers whose babies were allowed to nurse until they wanted to stop, we have never detected any signs of unusual dependence upon the mother. Actually they are *more* independent and in fact develop their independence earlier, in many cases.

If we had ever seen any signs to the contrary, we might take a second look at the theory that "all babies should be completely weaned by nine months" (or one year, or whatever). But it has been our experience, and that of many other mothers, that these little ones who have been allowed to grow out of nursing gradually and at their own pace, without anxiety or prematurity on the part of the mother, are happier, more independent little people.

Let the Baby Do It

So our suggestion is—let the baby do it. In this, as in everything else, you release, but you do not reject. You will, of course, be helping him along. Once he is eating a variety of solid foods you will find him losing interest in nursing, one feeding at a time. Taking his cue, just skip that nursing next time around, unless he has clearly changed his mind. In other words, you don't *refuse* the breast, but you don't *offer* it at that feeding either, unless the baby asks for it or your breast is uncomfortably full. You'll find that as he reaches the end of his first year, nursing will have gradually dwindled down to just naptime or bedtime. Of course, if he is ill or has hurt himself, nursing is not only a wonderful comfort to him but a godsend indeed to his mother. Many a wakeful night of floor-walking has been averted because a feverish, unhappy toddler has been taken in with mommy and allowed to nurse himself back to sleep. And though a sick child may steadfastly refuse all other food or be unable to keep it down, he will seldom refuse the breast or be unable to tolerate breast milk, which thus supplies nourishment and fluids as well as comfort to the ailing little one.

Oftentimes the older baby wants to nurse only because

he has nothing else more interesting to do. You will find that if you devote your attention to your baby-child not only when he is nursing but in other ways as well, his demand to be nursed lessens. Fifteen minutes or so occasionally devoted primarily to him will make him very happy. Even an eighteen-month-old enjoys being read to or just talked to, not in an absent-minded, distracted way while you are preoccupied with other things, but with your whole attention centered on him. Get down to his level. Sit on the floor with him. Let him know that you are very much interested in him and his activities. He will respond gratefully and joyously and become a remarkably independent little boy or girl sooner than you think.

If you should become pregnant again while nursing, there is no need to become concerned. You have several months in which to let the baby taper off gradually. During this time double up on your personal attention to the baby. Spend more time with him in other ways to compensate for ending what has been a happy breastfeeding relationship and to show him that the new kinds of relationship with him as an older baby are fun too.

Even though pregnancy may lead you to start weaning the baby a little earlier than you might if you were waiting for him to show definite signs of readiness, you still handle it in the same relaxed way. You leave out one nursing at a time, cutting out no more than one a week and never being *inflexible* about it, especially if the little one is ill or upset for some reason. You'll use your ingenuity to make the time at which you are omitting the nursing warm and happy in other ways. And remember, there's no hurry. Abrupt weaning is always to be avoided; it can be emotionally harmful to the baby and can lead to painful engorgement and even a breast infection in the mother. Whether you or the baby is taking the initiative, be easy and gradual about it. At some point along the line, your tactful encouragement will blend imperceptibly with the baby's own natural inclination to taper off. That way, the milk supply will diminish slowly but surely and finally disappear. And as baby nurses less and less, he will be discovering the joys of new relationships with you—sharing little jokes, play-acting with toys, enjoying simple songs, exploring together the wonderful out-of-doors (which is the baby's-eye view of the back yard or the walk to the grocery store).

Occasionally after being completely weaned a toddler might suddenly ask to be nursed again. (This sometimes happens when the new baby arrives.) Don't be afraid to take care of his need. It will only be temporary. Most likely, instead of nursing he will giggle and slide off your lap, reassured by your awareness of his need and your willingness to go along with it.

And do, do learn to turn a deaf ear to the dismal chorus of meddlesome voices: "You mean he's *still* nursing?" . . . . "Isn't he toilet trained yet?" . . . . "He's *still* waking up at night? Tsk, tsk, tsk!" This is *your* child, and you are doing what you know is best for him. You are cheerfully aware that you can't *worry* him out of his baby habits; that it's part of the fine art of mothering not to push him faster than he's able to go, just as it's part of the fine art of mothering not to hold him back when he's ready. It is when we impatiently try to force *our* pace on our little ones that we run into resistance, rebellion, and difficulty in later life. No matter what we do, or don't do, as the child grows he will eventually learn to use the toilet; learn acceptable table manners through good example; sleep like a rock all night; and also give up nursing. We can satisfy ourselves with the good thought that at his own pace he has grown out of each of his baby habits and is more secure because of our sensitive respect for him as an individual.

To sum up our philosophy of weaning, we repeat: Let the baby do it. Let him nurse until he wants to stop. Be sure that, when he is ready, he will "graduate." Weaning is a personal affair. It should take into consideration primarily the needs of the baby as recognized by the observant mother. You see, your baby has his own individual growth pattern in this respect, too. He is different from all other babies as to when he will cut his first tooth, when he will sit up by himself, and when he will walk and talk. Your baby may need the special kind of mothering he gets from breastfeeding for a longer time than someone else's baby. You, his mother, know and understand that need best because you have cared for him since he was born. With the special kind of love a mother has for her baby, you can sense his needs better than anyone else. This is why each baby has his own individual mother and is not turned out on an assembly-line, mass-produced basis.

DISCIPLINE

Why do we speak of discipline at all here, in writing of mere babies? Primarily because too often parents tend to jump the gun in this matter or to misunderstand it entirely. Discipline is a much-maligned word. It has a rather stern, unhappy, military connotation for most of us. We often come to associate it with punishment and deprivations. Yet this should not be the case. Discipline really refers to that guidance which we as parents lovingly give our children to help them do the right things for the right reasons; to help them grow into secure, happy, and loving persons able to step out into the world with confidence in their own ability to succeed in whatever they set out to do.

The laws of a new baby's growth are operating so strongly that all you can do is cooperate with them or frustrate them; he can't at an early age understand or follow laws imposed from without. If you are friendly and cooperative as he follows his own growth patterns, he can lay a sound foundation for further growth. If you are continually trying to force him into a pattern of your own making, or one prescribed by another, you will confuse him and perhaps interfere badly with his emotional development. "Just as the twig is bent, the tree's inclined," the wise old saying goes. Its moral is not to force the child this way or that, but to let him follow his own inner growth patterns in the image of the good values of the parents whom he learns to love. Then the tree will be straight and tall.

When we willingly, happily, lovingly nurse our babies, we are sensitive to their needs and instinctively meet them as fully as we can. A good beginning! The infant is ready to grow into childhood.

As the baby-child grows, he will necessarily need guidance, instruction, and sometimes correction to learn the ways

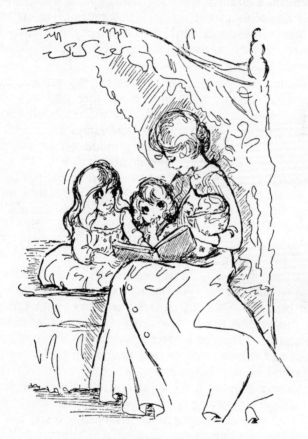

Discipline is loving guidance

of our world. If the foundation of secure love has been laid when he was a baby, he *wants* to act in socially approved ways and really needs little more than example and gentle suggestion to do so. We still have to respect his growth patterns, and not ask of him more than he is capable of giving at his stage of development, but we can and should give some direction to his inexperience. However, there is no sharp break in our ways of guiding our child's development. Abrupt weaning, sudden decisions to "train" the child to do this or that (as if he were a puppy) are unreasonable and can be harmful. Certainly spanking and slapping have no place in true discipline of the infant. They more often reflect the immaturity, impatience, and frustrations of the mother. What we resent in the unsuccessful school teacher, we should resent in ourselves.

While most people tend to respect the growth pattern of the small infant, the eighteen-monther or two-year-old toddler is another story. When little fingers reach for electric plugs, pennies go to mouths, and lamps are tossed over, thoughts of stern discipline and spankings rear their ugly heads. Of course, we can't permit utter chaos in a house, or unrestricted freedom that could be dangerous. But in handling these situations, we need to recognize that another growth pattern is showing itself. The toddler is now discovering the world around him, so he (and some more than others) wants to touch, feel, and take apart what he sees. He is just a normal two-year-old private eye, investigating everything and tracking it down. Punishing him will only frustrate his curious streak. Let him go; but be careful of what you leave within his reach. Not all children are alike; with some it is enough to caution them a few times about a forbidden object. If the child can learn to respect a few taboos without nagging or scolding from the mother, and frustration on his part, then this method is fine. Usually it is wiser to remove dangerous or breakable objects from sight entirely. In the case of a really dangerous situation, the mother should allow herself the full emotional expression of reasonable fears; the child will gradually adopt these fears of real dangers and avoid them.

In any case, keep an eye on him, for his own safety. Pediatric experts who have carefully studied accident patterns in the very young child state that it is only when a child has reached the age of approximately three that you can *begin* to teach him how to protect himself. Until that age he can only be protected by the ever-watching eyes of his elders, and it's up to you to make sure the eyes are there.

In discipline of any sort, as with the care you've been giving your baby right from the start, consistency is a key word. Know how you plan to act in a given situation and stick to it. Say "No" as seldom as possible. (Saying "No" often is what teaches a child to say "No" more often than "Yes," which is not the road to true discipline.) When you do say "No," let him know you mean it, calmly, firmly, and cheerfully. It usually works better just to pick him up, with a cheerful hug, and remove him from the source of trouble, drawing his attention casually to some other fascinating object or activity. *Little* babies distract rather easily. As they get older, you need to use more finesse, but an ounce of distraction is still worth a pound of exhorting.

Notice that word "usually" in the last paragraph. How often we use that word, and others like it, in this book! Every time we do, it's really a reminder of the one main point we keep emphasizing: babies are individuals, and you can't lay down hard-and-fast rules for all of them. In this matter of discipline too, if you have the intimate understanding of your little one which the breastfeeding relationship fosters, and if you are clear in your own mind about the real nature of discipline, you can safely follow your own instincts as parents.

TOILET HABITS

When will your child have his toilet habits under control? This varies, like everything else, with the individual child. Some children acquire control of the sphincter, or "hold-back" muscles sooner than others. The timing is a matter of no real importance. Parental intervention is perhaps more likely to delay it than hasten it. Often, enough bowel control to prevent "accidents" most of the time comes toward the end of the second year; the same degree of daytime bladder control, about a year later. "Sleeping dry" is usually last of all. But there is considerable individual variation. Your part is simply to give your little one friendly encouragement and to let him observe from time to time how older children and grownups manage the details. He'll do the rest.

In this, as in other aspects of growth, you let him know

how pleased and proud you are about his accomplishments; but don't make too big a production of this either, or the inevitable lapses might cause him more concern than they should. Treat "mistakes," when they occur, with casual sympathy and, especially as the child gets older, help him save face by quick and unobtrusive disposal of the evidence.

Staying dry all night happens when his bladder gets large enough to hold the amount of urine that accumulates during the night. Even after your child is able to start and stop urinating at will when he is awake, his bladder will still empty automatically at night when it becomes overfull—a wise precaution of Nature's. One of the things that helps the bladder grow large enough to hold the night urine is the child's occasional holding of the urine somewhat *past* the time when he feels the urge to void during his waking hours; this stretches the bladder gently. You can see then that an overanxious mother who watches her toddler narrowly and rushes him to the toilet every two hours, or every time he shows signs of needing to urinate, may actually be delaying the time when he is able to sleep dry through the night.

However, your young child will normally from time to time become very absorbed in what he is doing. We usually describe this as playing, but it is really working at learning about the world, about his own abilities, about other people and his relation to them. He may become so absorbed that he won't let himself be conscious of the growing feeling of bladder fullness, sometimes until too late to avoid an "accident." If the situation is one in which this might cause embarrassment or property damage, and you notice his absent-minded contortions in time, you might offer a tactful reminder. But taking himself to the bathroom is essentially *his* business. Actually, in waiting a while sometimes and unconsciously letting the accumulating urine stretch his bladder a little, he is tending to the business of growing better than if you interfere.

Of course, it's necessary for a while to lend a hand with such things as "wiping" and washing hands afterward, but this help can be given in a casual way. You take the same friendly interest in his comfort in this respect as you do in other ways, and continue to help as needed until he gradually takes over for himself the socially approved routines of toileting, with the same casual attitude he has learned from you. Easy does it.

THE HEART OF THE MATTER

What we have been saying in this chapter is simply this: the same principles you follow in feeding your child may well be the models for your handling of all aspects of his development.

When your child is born, you devote yourself unstintingly to meeting his needs; you nurse him when he is hungry and hold him snug and warm and close as long as he needs and likes it. As he grows, he wants less snuggle and more sociability; you prop him up in the midst of the family from time to time and go about your business of cooking or whatever—never getting too far away, so that when his brief spurt of "independence" has spent itself, you can welcome him back to the haven of mother's arms. As the days and weeks and months go by, he becomes more independent in other ways; he starts eating solid foods and does not nurse so long or so often. Soon he not only accepts the food you put in his mouth, but picks up bits of food to bring them to his mouth himself. And one day, lo: he is feeding himself, handling a spoon with dignity and aplomb, albeit with occasional spectacular messes. Now he is drinking milk from a cup and taking no more than a friendly nightcap from the breast, except when trouble with teething, or a bump from adventuring, or a cold coming on, makes him seek the solace of the same old familiar comfort. You are still there when he needs you. There is never an abrupt withdrawal of your love as expressed first through the warmth and closeness of nursing and later in other ways. Secure in knowing that he can retreat for a bit into babyhood if he wants to, he ventures further and further into childhood, and finally (all too soon, it seems in retrospect), he isn't a baby any more, but a big boy; he eats at the family table and enjoys the family meals. In the not too distant future, he will be trudging off to school with his lunchbox. And far down the years you catch a misty glimpse of him as he struggles with those first uncertain meals prepared by his young bride, and later still as he watches with pride as his son gets *his* good beginning in life at her breast.

We hope that in these few pages we have been able to give you a perspective or point of view about the way in which we believe the start in life you give your child through breastfeeding can lead to disciplined maturity. With your understanding guidance, your child will grow from dependence to independence gradually, and always with the love that is his birthright, and the great need of our world.

Booklist

Most mothers will want to do more reading about pre-natal care, child care, and nutrition than we have included in this book about breastfeeding. You may even want to read more about breastfeeding. The following books and other materials are recommended; where our experience differs in any important respect from certain parts of a book, we say so. Prices of course are subject to change. (See "Where to Obtain Books and Pamphlets," p. 146.)

A word of warning: especially as you get into the child care area, read as much as you like, but always remember to rely *most* on your own motherly instincts, taking into account your own and your family's particular personality differences, likes and dislikes, and so on. Don't try to do everything "by the book." Just relax and be a mother.

PRENATAL

A Baby Is Born, Maternity Center Association, 64 pp., hardcover, $3.95. LLLI.

> This book is designed to help not only mothers but every-one to learn the basic facts about human reproduction. The many illustrations are mainly diagrams and photographs of the famous Dickinson-Belski sculptures which also appear in the Center's much larger, better-known BIRTH ATLAS. The book shows not only the baby's development, but what happens to the mother's internal organs as the uterus in-creases in size. The text is brief, but adequate and interesting.

OTHER SOURCES

There is excellent information about prenatal care in the books on natural childbirth listed under "Childbirth," and in *The Family Book of Child Care*, listed under "Child Care." The Children's Bureau of the U. S. Department of Health, Education, and Welfare puts out a pamphlet called *Prenatal Care* (15¢); order from Superintend-ent of Documents, U. S. Government Printing Office, Washington D. C. 20402.

CHILDBIRTH

Methods of Childbirth, Constance A. Bean. Garden City, N.Y.: Doubleday & Co., 1972. 210 pp. $6.95. LLLI.

An unbiased, readable analysis of current trends in childbirth, explaining in detail the different "methods" of prepared childbirth —Lamaze, Read, etc. Good brief discussions of the mother-doctor relationship, drugs and anesthesia (pro and con), and childbirth education classes.

Emergency Childbirth, Gregory J. White, M.D. Franklin Park, Ill: Police Training Foundation, 1958. 62 pp. $3.00. LLLI.

The standard manual for policemen and others who may have to assist when the mother can't make it to the hospital, or the doctor to her, in time. Excellent reading for prospective parents because of the clear, well-illustrated description of the birth process by Dr. White.

Husband-Coached Childbirth, Robert A. Bradley, M.D. New York: Harper & Row, 1965. 208 pp. $5.50. LLLI.

The author, a Denver obstetrician, depicts the primary duty of the doctor as prenatal teacher of husband and wife, and the husband's role as physical conditioning coach. We disagree rather strongly with three things in the book: the author's views on routine use of episiotomy, his absolute opposition to home delivery, and his advocating a regular night out for the mother without her baby, from the time the baby is a couple of weeks old. Otherwise an excellent book on childbirth.

The Experience of Childbirth, Sheila Kitzinger. 3rd ed.; Baltimore, Md.: Penguin Books, 1972. 280 pp. Paperback $1.95. LLLI.

Warm, woman's-eye view of childbirth. Explains in detail the physiology of pregnancy, development of fetus, and actual process of normal labor. A mother of four, the author claims there are very few women who cannot bear their children consciously, and with great joy. Her teaching is derived in part from the methods of Dick-Read and in part from Lamaze and Vellay. The greatest emphasis is on emotional preparation and the importance of the husband during labor and delivery.

Childbirth without Fear, Grantly Dick-Read, M.D. New York: Harper & Row. 4th ed., rev. & ed. by Helen Wessel and Harlan F. Ellis, M.D., 1972. 420 pp., hardcover only, $7.95. LLLI. 2d ed., 1970 [last revision by Dr. Dick-Read]. 384 pp., paperback only, 95¢. LLLI.

Dr. Dick-Read was the pioneer in the field of natural childbirth. Always in demand, his trailblazing book is still available as he revised and enlarged it (paperback only). In the new hardcover edition it has been reorganized and "Americanized," with some new material added.

The Natural Childbirth Primer, Grantly Dick-Read, M.D. New York: Harper & Row, 1956. 52 pp. $2.50. LLLI.

Clear and simple, it explains the basic principles of childbirth as a normal natural womanly function.

Childbirth without Pain, Pierre Vellay and others. Translated by Denise Lloyd. New York: E. P. Dutton & Co., 1960. 216 pp. $6.95. ICEA.

This book provides some of the basic training lectures on the psychoprophylactic method of childbirth. Dr. Vellay is an associate of Dr. Lamaze. The first half is rather technical and not easy to read, but the second half consists of reports from new mothers who tell of their birth experiences using this method. The photos should convince even the most skeptical that it is possible to give birth joyously.

Six Practical Lessons for an Easier Childbirth, by Elisabeth Bing, R.P.T. New York: Bantam Books, 1969. 128 pp., paperback, $1.00. LLLI.

An easy-to-read book of instructions in the Lamaze Method of childbirth preparation, it is designed for the couple who cannot attend classes and emphasizes the husband's role in the preparation as well as during the actual labor.

BREASTFEEDING

Nursing your Baby, Karen Pryor. New York: Harper & Row, 1973. 289 pp., paperback, $1.50. LLLI.

Based on considerable research by the author, plus experience as the mother of three. Comprehensive descriptions of how the breasts function and the content of human milk. Good practical hints too, in a lively, readable style.

The Tender Gift: Breastfeeding, Dana Raphael. Englewood Cliffs, N.J.: Prentice-Hall, Inc., 1973. 200 pp., hardcover, $6.95. LLLI.

Dr. Raphael, an anthropologist, gives a fascinating account of breastfeeding in many cultures and among animal groups. Most importantly, she develops the concept of "mothering the mother," emphasizing the special help and support which women need following pregnancy and childbirth as they get used to their new role and become sensitive to the needs of their babies.

Abreast of the Times, R. M. Applebaum, M.D. Miami, Fla.; 1969. 88 pp. Softcover. $2.50. LLLI.

Dr. Applebaum believes very firmly in the tremendous advantages of breastfeeding and does not hesitate to say so.

Breastfeeding and Natural Child Spacing, Sheila Kippley. New York: Harper & Row, 1974. 197 pp., hardcover, $6.95. LLLI.

A well-documented study, highly recommended for those interested in this aspect of breastfeeding, as well as for all who want to understand the values of a close mother-baby relationship.

CHILD CARE

There are so many good books on child care, it's hard to make a selection. You may already have one you swear by. If so, by all means hang onto it—but pass up the pages about making formula.

The Family Book of Child Care, Niles Newton, Ph.D. New York: Harper & Row, 1957. 477 pp. $8.95. LLLI.

Pregnancy, childbirth, and breastfeeding are much more than clinically outlined in this book. The relaxed attitude of the author, mother of four, is contagious and makes the tremendous vocation of parenthood seem just a little less overwhelming. Certain sections seem geared more to the bottle-fed baby, and the section on weaning is not in accord with LLL recommendations. It's a good baby shower gift.

Teaching Montessori in the Home, Elizabeth G. Hainstock, Maryland: Random House, 1968. 117 pp., hardcover, $6.95. LLLI.

A very readable book, showing how a child's best teacher (his mother) can adapt the Montessori principles to her children in her home. Excellent bibliography gives sources for more information. Construction of any tools required is described, using materials available in the home. Patterns for letters, numbers, and symbols are included.

The Child Under Six, James L. Hymes, Jr. Englewood Cliffs, N.J.: Prentice-Hall, Inc., 1966. 342 pp. $6.95. LLLI.

Beautiful concepts of the young child's need for love. We have only a few minor disagreements with the book, one being the author's favoring nursery school from age three. (Too young for most little ones, we think.) Also, he feels a baby under six months can easily be left at home and won't know the difference. On the whole, an excellent, warm, and inspiring book.

Babies Are Human Beings, C. Anderson Aldrich, M.D. and Mary M. Aldrich. 2nd ed.; New York: Macmillan Co., 1954. 122 pp. Collier paperback edition, 95¢.

One of the "classics" in this field. The hardbound edition, now out of print, is available in most libraries; and fortunately a paperback edition has now been issued. The authors discuss the growth and development of babies from birth. They recognize a "dynamic quality"—a force within the baby and child which causes him to make continued efforts to assert himself despite the obstacles and frustrations placed in his way by a restrictive society.

The Rights of Infants, Margaret A. Ribble. 2nd ed.; New York: Columbia Press, 1965. 148 pp. $6.00; paperback 95¢. ICEA.

Another classic on the basic needs of babies which has helped to swing child care away from old "don't-pick-them-up-or-you'll-spoil-them" theories.

COOKBOOKS

Mother's in the Kitchen, edited by Roberta Johnson. Franklin Park, Illinois: La Leche League International, 1971. 228 pp. Softcover. $4.00. LLLI.

The League's own cookbook, made up of recipes submitted and family-tested by League mothers interested in good nutrition as well as tastiness, economy, and ease of preparation. Includes some basic principles of nutrition which the appetizing woman-to-woman recipes make it easy to practice.

The Natural Baby Food Cookbook, Margaret Elizabeth Kenda and Phyllis S. Williams. New York: Avon Books, 1973. 168 pp., paperback, 95¢. LLLI.

The authors have carefully researched current nutritional findings and adapted them to guidelines for feeding the family. There are suggestions for feeding allergic, finicky, or sick children, following the same good nutritional guidelines. Some interesting recipes are included.

PAMPHLETS

Enjoy Your Child—Ages 1, 2, and 3, James L. Hymes, Jr. Public Affairs Pamphlet No. 141. Public Affairs Pamphlets, 381 Park Ave., South, New York, N. Y. 10016. 25¢.

Breastfeeding, Audrey Palm Riker, Public Affairs Pamphlet No. 353S. 16 pp. 25¢. LLLI.

Breast Feeding Your Baby. Children's Bureau Folder No. 8, 1965. Superintendent of Documents, U. S. Government Printing Office, Washington, D. C. 20402. 27 pp. 10¢.

The Uniqueness of Human Milk, edited by D. B. and E. F. P. Jelliffe. Reprinted from *The American Journal of Clinical Nutrition,* 24 (1971): 967-1024. $1.75. LLLI.

On Discipline: A Symposium, Nancy Stanton, Jalelah Fraley, Dolores Cuthbertson, and Judy Good. Reprinted from *La Leche League News,* 15 (1973), 33-44. 25¢. LLLI.

More Than Sandpaper Letters: Montessori in the Home, Doma Petrutis. Reprinted from *Child and Family,* 8 (1969). 16 pp. 50¢. LLLI.

The Modern Management of Successful Breast Feeding, R. M. Applebaum, M.D. Reprinted from *Pediatric Clinics of North America,* 17 (1970): 203-225. 25¢. LLLI.

See also La Leche League pamphlets listed on p. 155.

WHERE TO OBTAIN BOOKS AND PAMPHLETS

Books can be purchased at or through your bookstore. Many of them are in your public library. Pamphlets can be ordered from the addresses listed. Some books and pamphlets can be purchased from La Leche League International (LLLI) or the International Childbirth Education Association (ICEA); when this is the case, the initials appear directly after the price. Publications ordered from LLLI or ICEA bring these organizations a small profit which helps them continue their services to mothers.

LLLI La Leche League International ICEA ICEA Supplies Center
     9616 Minneapolis Ave.   1414 N.W. 85th St.
     Franklin Park, Ill. 60131   Seattle, Wash. 98117

About This Book and Its Authors

We have written this book especially for you.

"You" are someone who wants to breastfeed her baby, a mother who wants to give her child the very best possible start in life.

Naturally, you will want to know who "we" are. Although all of us are mothers who enjoy nursing our babies and who want to encourage you and give you the benefit of our know-how, we have each had different experiences in gaining confidence in ourselves as nursing mothers.

So we would like to introduce ourselves individually to you, telling you a little about ourselves and our families.

MARIAN TOMPSON, the petite president of La Leche League, who combines soft-spoken femininity with effective leadership, is the wife of Clement, a research engineer, and mother of Melanie, Deborah, Allison, Laurel, Sheila, and Brian. Melanie was nursed for six months despite very little information on breastfeeding. But with each of the next two babies Marian thought her milk was disappearing after a few weeks and put them on the bottle. All it took was an experienced, encouraging doctor and the example of other nursing mothers to enable Marian to completely breastfeed her next three children a year or more.

MARY WHITE, in charge of research for the League, is married to Gregory J., a physician, and is the mother of Joseph, William, Margaret, Catherine, Anne, Regina, Michael,

Mary Cecilia, and Clare Marie. With her husband in the Army, Mary didn't find breastfeeding easy that first time eighteen years ago. Too many supplementary bottles resulted in her "losing her milk," and this soon meant the end of nursing. Through determination, and with the help of her husband, the second baby was completely breastfed as were all the rest of the children. Mary, relaxed and easygoing, is also proof that a mother usually can and should continue to nurse if she has a breast infection. She had one which had to be incised and drained, yet all worked out well and with a minimum of difficulty.

EDWINA FROEHLICH, articulate secretary of the League, is the understanding voice that answers the League's home-office phone. She is the wife of John, an internal revenue officer, and mother of Paul, David, and Peter. Edwina was thirty-five years old when her first baby was born. Aside from a little difficulty with sore nipples, she had no trouble nursing Paul, being fortunate in having both the practical help of her doctor and the moral support of her husband and her mother. Each of Edwina's three sons gained their first twenty pounds or so solely on breast milk and never used a bottle.

MARY ANN KERWIN was formerly our librarian and is now head of six flourishing groups in Denver. Youthful, enthusiastic Mary Ann is the wife of Thomas, an attorney, and mother of Thomas Jr., Edward, Joseph (now in heaven), Gregory, and Mary Elizabeth. Mary Ann had to work almost a week with her first baby before he really took to nursing. Still she did not use any supplementary bottles during that time and subsequently found complete breastfeeding easy with the other children.

BETTY WAGNER, our treasurer, wife of Robert, a machinist, is the mother of Gail, Robert, Wayne, Mary, Margaret, Dorothea, and Helen. It was Betty's mother who strongly encouraged Betty to breastfeed when Gail was born, and her husband quietly supported the idea. Gail was colicky, and a few supplementary bottles were tried. When these proved to be of no help, Betty calmly and with her own characteristically deft and practical approach went back to complete nursing and the use of a pacifier. All her babies have been nursed nine months or more.

VIOLA LENNON, smart and smart-looking, is married to William, an attorney and labor organizer, and is the mother of Elizabeth, Mark, Melissa, Rebecca, Matthew, Catherine, Charlotte, and Martin. All but one of the Lennon babies were completely nursed, but Vi's real "claim to fame" is her breastfeeding of the twins, Catherine and Charlotte. Wakeful and fussy as an infant, Cathy nursed every two hours and weaned herself at eleven months. Sleepy Charlotte nursed much less often but continued until she was fourteen months old. The rest of us feel *we* could have done just as well with twins, but we have to admit that Vi's unruffled poise and laconic humor were useful qualities to have in that situation.

MARY ANN CAHILL, for several years editor of the LLL NEWS, is the imaginative, red-haired wife of Charles, an accountant, and mother of Robert Jerome (who joined the family when he was two and a half years old), Elizabeth, Timothy, Teresa, Mary, Joseph, and Margaret. Mary Ann has never had the engorgement or leaking of the breasts that so many mothers experience. With her first baby, this led to many doubts as to whether or not she really had enough milk, and as a result Elizabeth was nursed only three months. But meeting a doctor with experience in helping nursing mothers enabled Mary Ann to completely breastfeed the rest of her children.

Seven mothers, seven personalities. Over forty breastfed babies, some now grown-up teen-agers on their way to college, some still "new and nursing." No two are alike, of course, even in the same family. But peaceful or bouncy, tall or short, lightning-quick or sleepy-slow, they all have one thing in common: they're all happy, friendly, and unusually healthy.

Some day they will all go their separate ways, each doing what he thinks best. Some day they may be raising families of their own, proudly and lovingly, giving each child a secure foundation in life, starting from the moment of birth and those happy months of breastfeeding. They will know that this heritage given them by their own parents is to be passed on from generation to generation.

So much for us and our families. Now a bit more about this book. We haven't put a lot of footnotes and references in it, because it isn't that kind of book. But you may like to know that we do have sound medical authority for the statements of fact we make. Also, our medical consultants have read the book and approve it. These consultants have many nursing mothers in their practices and are familiar at first-hand with the problems involved. Our chief claim to authenticity, though, rests on our experiences with our own babies and with the babies of thousands of other mothers whose experiences we have been privileged to share.

If you have a practical problem about breastfeeding, we invite you to ask us—and we do mean this. (See the following section for a description of La Leche League and how it operates.) If you have a medical problem, you will naturally ask your doctor.

We want to acknowledge, with heartfelt thanks, the help and encouragement of Dr. Herbert Ratner, Dr. Gregory J. White, Dr. Niles Newton, Dr. E. Robbins Kimball, Dr. Frank Howard Richardson, the late Dr. Grantly Dick-Read, Mrs. John Gayle Aiken, the late Mildred Hatch, and Mrs. Margaret Gamper, R.N. Any deficiencies in this book are in spite of their kindly interest and suggestions.

We are also grateful for professional help to artist Joy Sidor, whose own happy baby was her lovely model; to Dorothy Vining, whose gifted pen was responsible for the chapter on the father's role in the family; and to Mary B. Carson, who edited the manuscript.

A special debt of gratitude is owed to the wonderful women whose enthusiastic competence in starting new La Leche groups in other communities has added immeasurably to the fund of experience on which we have drawn, as well as to those in our own community who have helped with much of the detail work.

About La Leche League

We, the seven author-mothers introduced in the preceding section, are a part of La Leche League, though in truth only a small part. It is time to tell about La Leche.

The founding League in Franklin Park is a non-sectarian, not-for-profit corporation. Everyone interested in breastfeeding is of interest to La Leche League. "La Leche," which is Spanish and is pronounced "La Lay-chay," means simply "The Milk."

Breastfeeding was a part of womanly concern and devotion in the earliest settlement in America. In 1598 in St. Augustine, Florida, a shrine was dedicated to the Mother of Christ under the title "Nuestra Senora de la Leche y Buen Parto," which translates freely, "Our Lady of Happy Delivery and Plentiful Milk," and is the source of the name we chose for our League.

We believe that La Leche—"The Milk"—is a name that is also meaningful to today's nursing mother. Breastfeeding gives the baby back to the mother. Her baby securely in her arms, she finds her motherly response, like her milk, is never measured, but ample.

Breastfeeding is a part of a womanly heritage, and it would naturally follow, in fact it seems almost inevitable, that mothers should initiate the revival in breastfeeding. Not that professional work and interest are not important. Repeatedly, new evidence of the superiority of breastfeeding is brought to light through medical research. The facts are substantial and impressive, though scientific and lengthy. But someone is needed to emphasize and interpret the facts; someone with an understanding of just what a new mother needs

151

to know. Someone must be handy to reassure and encourage her. Why not another nursing mother? She would have understanding and enthusiasm and, let us hope, a simple touch.

Certainly the beginnings of La Leche League were simple. Mary White and Marian Tompson sat at a picnic, a family-type picnic, complete with babies. They talked about babies and breastfeeding, the joy of both, and deplored the fact that many mothers who wanted to nurse their babies did not succeed, for want of help. "Couldn't we, and some of the other nursing mothers we know, help?"

So the League began. The other five of us joined, and several doctors well-versed in breastfeeding agreed to stand by as medical consultants. We set out to learn all we could about breastfeeding. We read books and medical publications, collected facts, examined old wives' tales, and shared experiences. When we summed it all up, again it was simple. Babies were meant to be breastfed, and they could be. We knew without a doubt.

In October, 1956, in a home in Franklin Park, Illinois, La Leche League held its first meeting. The group was made up of the seven of us and several of our friends who were expecting babies; the purpose, to give them the benefit of what we had learned and experienced. We hoped that they, too, could have the joy and satisfaction of nursing their babies. And this pattern of a small, informal group of mothers, meeting to learn and to exchange experiences, has been League practice ever since.

But how the League has grown! We had no idea there were so many women eager to nurse their babies. The Franklin Park group has expanded into fifty-five groups in the Chicago area and over twelve hundred more throughout the United States and in fifteen other countries. They all follow more or less the same pattern: a series of meetings held in a home, covering about the same ground as this book, and giving the mothers a chance to talk with other expectant or nursing mothers, share their experiences and be on the giving or receiving end of advice about problems that might come up. In some areas there is a special meeting, "For Fathers Only." Also, because personal contact with other nursing mothers is so important when you are new at the womanly art, we always encourage new mothers to visit, write, or telephone experienced League mothers if they have questions or

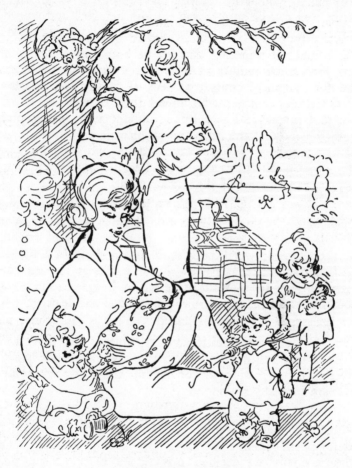

It all started at a picnic

need reassurance. A toll call is less costly than formula and bottles.

Of course, it wouldn't be humanly possible for the seven of us to talk or write to all the thousands of mothers who have heard of La Leche League and ask for help in getting started with breastfeeding. For one thing, we all put the needs of our own families first. Providentially, the number of experienced and enthusiastic mothers willing to help keeps growing. If you write us, you may be hearing from one of them: you can be sure that we know her well and consider her eminently well qualified as an experienced nursing mother.

Sometimes a mother asks for help with a medical problem. First and foremost we tell her to check with her doctor about it. Then, of course, we tell her of the experiences of other nursing mothers who, under their doctors' care, were able and encouraged to continue nursing with similar problems. But most of the time, the problems aren't medical, and all that is needed is the practical advice and encouragement of another mother; this any of the League mothers are happy to give, at any hour of the day or night.

You can see that the League is by no means an impersonal, highly organized association. Rather, we are most informal, trying to keep everything on the basis of friendly conversations between mothers. You can think of La Leche League, if you like, as a woman with a baby in her arms and a smile on her face, proud of herself and eager to share with you the wealth of all she has experienced and learned.

It should probably be said that we make little effort to persuade mothers to breastfeed their babies if they don't want to. As a practical matter, we already have our hands happily more than full passing on our nursing know-how to mothers who are earnestly seeking it.

This book is really the La Leche League manual, developed originally for mothers too far away from a group to attend meetings. For some time it circulated in a planographed edition; finally, we decided to revise and expand it and publish it in regular book form.

Besides the manual, we publish a cookbook, MOTHER'S IN THE KITCHEN (see page 145), and the bimonthly LA LECHE LEAGUE NEWS, in which we exchange news and views and practical mother-to-mother suggestions. The NEWS also contains occasional book reviews and reports on medical research related to breastfeeding. Subscription price is $2.75 a year, $7.50 for three years; Canada and Mexico $3.25 a year, other countries $3.75 a year.

In addition, we have such pamphlets as:

Why Breastfeed Your Baby?

For mothers. Tells about La Leche League and hits the high points of the reasons for breastfeeding. #101-Free.

How the Nurse Can Help the Breastfeeding Mother

For nurses. Practical suggestions on how nurses can help mothers get started breastfeeding, what advise to give them about continuing when they leave the hospital, and how to refer them to La Leche League if they need more help. #118-50¢ per copy.

When You Breastfeed Your Baby

For new mothers. Discusses briefly the how-to of breastfeeding in the hospital and during the early weeks at home and refers to this manual and to La Leche for additional information. #124-10¢ per copy.

One copy of each of these pamphlets and a copy of La Leche League News will be sent for eighty-five cents in coin or postage. (ask for #97).

Maybe you would like to be a member of La Leche League. The dues are $8.00 a year ($8.50 outside U.S.A.); this includes a subscription to LA LECHE LEAGUE NEWS. If you attend a group, you pay your dues to the group treasurer. If you are not attending a group, send your dues direct to La Leche League International with a note saying you want to be a member. Whether you're a member or not, remember that interested women (and babies) are always welcome at LLL groups meetings, and that *anyone* can write or call us for advice or encouragement about breastfeeding, at any time.

Our address is:

LA LECHE LEAGUE INTERNATIONAL
FRANKLIN PARK, ILLINOIS 60131

Even if you never get in touch with us, we hope it helps you to know that all over the country womanly women are breastfeeding their babies and that advice and encouragement are available to you if you need them in learning this most womanly art.

Index